EMBRACING THE JOURNEY

A CAREGIVER'S SURVIVAL GUIDE TO LATE-STAGE DEMENTIA

ROSALIND BAKER-WARREN

TABLE OF CONTENTS

Introduction   5

1. UNDERSTANDING LATE STAGE DEMENTIA   13
   Changes in Moderate (Stage 5) Dementia   14
   Dementia Stage 5: Moderately Severe Cognitive
   Decline   15
   Cognitive Changes in Moderately Severe (Stage 6)
   Dementia   17
   Emotional and Behavioral Aspects   19
   Physical Changes and Care Needs   23
   Palliative Care and Pain Management   24
   Creating a Safe and Supportive Environment   24
   Caregiver Self-Care and Emotional Well-Being   25
   Coping With Grief and Loss   27
   Segue   30

2. PROVIDING PERSON-CENTERED CARE   31
   Understanding Person-Centered Care   32
   Benefits of Person-Centered Care   35
   The Royal Melbourne Hospital Case Study   36
   Implementing Person-Centered Care Practices   36
   Individualized Care Plans and Decision-Making   39
   Creating a Comforting and Supportive Environment   40
   Promoting Autonomy and Decision-Making   41
   Segue   42

3. COMMUNICATION TECHNIQUES AND
   STRATEGIES   45
   Understanding Communication Changes in Late-
   Stage Dementia   46
   Nonverbal Communication and Body Language   48
   Emotional and Sensory Communication   50
   Effective Communication Strategies   53
   Overcoming Communication Challenges   57
   Collaborating With Healthcare Professionals   58
   Segue   59

4. MANAGING CHALLENGING BEHAVIORS   61
Understanding Challenging Behaviors in Late-Stage
Dementia   62
Segue   69

5. NUTRITION AND HYDRATION IN LATE-STAGE
DEMENTIA   73
Understanding the Challenges of Eating and
Drinking in Late-Stage Dementia   74
Strategies for Promoting Nutritional Intake   77
Collaborating With Healthcare Professionals and
Caregivers   84
Support for Caregivers   85
Segue   86

6. LEGAL AND FINANCIAL PLANNING FOR
CAREGIVERS   87
Legal Planning for Caregivers   88
Financial Planning for Caregivers   92
Seeking Professional Assistance and Resources   96
Segue   99

7. RESOURCES AND SUPPORT SYSTEMS FOR
CAREGIVERS   101
Caregiver Support Organizations and Programs   103
Professional Support Services   110
Mental Health Support for Caregivers   115
Additional Resources and Strategies   116
Practical Resources for Daily Caregiving   121
Segue   123

8. END-OF-LIFE CONSIDERATIONS AND
PALLIATIVE CARE   125
Understanding End-of-Life in Late-Stage Dementia   126
Emotional and Psychological Considerations   131
Principles and Practices of Palliative Care   133
End-of-Life Decision-Making and Bereavement
Support   135

Conclusion   141
References   143

INTRODUCTION

Those with dementia are still people and they still have stories and they still have character and they're all individuals and they're all unique. And they just need to be interacted with on a human level.

— CAREY MULLIGAN

As a caregiver, know that you are fulfilling a much-needed position in your loved one's life. Life may get difficult, but you need to know that there are rewarding moments, humorous moments, and moments that will forever live in your memory.

This handbook will help you through any stumbling blocks you may have. You need to know that, statistically, you are not alone. A study by Brodaty and Donkin (2019) estimated that there are more than 30 million dementia sufferers in the world who need help from carers; in America, it is estimated that 75% of caregivers are directly related to the person needing the care either by family ties or by friendship.

CASE STUDIES

In order to help you feel comfortable in your role as a caregiver, let's look at some case studies. For security purposes, only initials will be used.

J. M.

J.M. is in the unenviable situation of caring for two people with dementia—her 95-year-old mother and her 40-year-old Down syndrome daughter. She has a unique way of looking at her situation. She finds joy in being able to care for them. She looks forward to the challenges and joy that each day brings. At the beginning of each day, she prepares herself as best she can, as every day is different and brings its own set of challenges and fun. It is all in the mindset.

She urges other caregivers to

- believe in themselves,
- have confidence that they are doing things the right way, and
- take time for yourself.

She works mainly from home, and other family members step in when she has to report to the office.

D. Q.

D.Q. cares for her nonagenarian grandmother. Her biggest challenge was ensuring that her grandmother was kept safe and healthy during COVID.

She urges other caregivers to

- make use of the many resources that are available, like associations dedicated to dementia, books, and internet sources,
- make sure that you have people you can count on to give you some relief from your duties, and
- get therapeutic help before it is needed.

B. S.

B. S. cares for her husband. She dances to an ever-changing beat, and steps are never guaranteed to be the same from one day to the next.

She urges carers to get some training or attend dementia workshops. In this way, a carer can meet with other carers and develop a support system outside their family or friends.

M. Z.

M. Z. cares for her husband, who has lived with dementia for almost 10 years. She feels that the most important thing is to keep the sufferer active. They joined a social dementia circle, which puts her in contact with other carers and gives her husband a new set of people to fraternize with in a fun-filled atmosphere. She makes sure to grab onto any resources that are useful.

P. H.

P.H. cared for her grandmother, who had dementia. When her grandmother died, P. H. was in denial about her mother, who was also showing signs of dementia. She soon came to realize, though, that her time of caring for a loved one with dementia was not over. She is now amazed at how different her mother is from her grandmother. Her grandmother was quiet, but her mother seeks to be busy all the time. As her mother was artistic, P. H. encourages her mother to draw and paint.

Types of Caregivers

As you can see, caregivers come from all walks of life and have various relationships with their loved ones. A couple of things can be learned from these stories:

- Don't forget self-care.
- Seek out resources to help you in your task.
- Get relief before the job drains you.

WHAT IS DEMENTIA?

There are many different types of dementia. The most well-known type is Alzheimer's disease. The beginnings of most dementias could start 20 years before the first symptoms make their appearance. Generally, dementias are split into seven stages, which are further grouped into three sections—early, middle, and late.

Early-stage dementia consists of three stages (1, 2, and 3). Middle-stage dementia consists of two stages (Stages 4 and 5). Late-stage dementia consists of two stages (6 and 7). Let's break these down:

Stage 1

You will not even be aware that dementia is working on the brain of your loved one.

Stage 2

Certain abilities are affected during this stage, but normal aging processes are very similar to dementia symptoms.

Stage 3

At this stage, it may be diagnosed as dementia, but it could still just reflect normal aging processes. Memory is affected now, and carers may interpret this as a warning that the loved one may be experiencing dementia.

Stage 4

During this stage, doctors can differentiate between normal aging and dementia symptoms. Personality changes may occur, and memory tends to worsen.

Stage 5

Loss of memory becomes more pronounced. They may forget family members' names or start to confuse one family member with another. This becomes worrying if the family name they remember belongs to a deceased relative, often a parent or a sibling.

The loved one will often appear confused and restless. They are prone to wander, which is concerning as they could easily get lost if allowed off the property. Restlessness increases as the day draws to a close, giving the term sundowning to this state.

Their problem-solving and logical abilities are reduced.

Stage 6

They will need help with basic daily activities like eating, dressing, and bathing. Incontinence becomes an issue. It is the stage where most caregivers will start to realize that full-time care is necessary.

Other factors become evident like:

- Your loved one shows some personality changes like aggression.
- They become anxious in situations that they have handled fine before.
- Memory loss is more evident, with stories and questions repeated within a short space of time.
- Insomnia increases.
- They are convinced that someone is out to hurt them or rob them.

Stage 7

This is the end stage of dementia.

- Memory is severely affected.
- Your loved one may lose the power of communicating as they cannot string words together in a coherent order.
- They will need help with everything, like moving from place to place and changing positions.
- They will have problems eating and may have to be fed by tubes.
- They will rest and sleep a lot during this stage.
- Total incontinence is evident.

SEGUE

This book focuses on late-stage dementia and will focus on stages 5 through 7. Chapter 1 will take you through understanding the late stages more completely.

UNDERSTANDING LATE STAGE DEMENTIA

Even If I can't cure, I can still care.

— SALLY P. KARIOTH RN, PHD (WHEELCHAIR-
BOUND)

You, as a caregiver, must be open to the fact that there will be challenges as you proceed through this journey with your loved one. It is going to be emotional at times, but there are rewards to be garnered along the way. Every now and then, some elements of your loved one will peek out.

In an emotional video, former ballerina Marta Cinta González Saldaña responded to the music of Swan Lake (Alzheimer's Research Association, 2020). She was wheelchair-bound, but eventually, the strains of the music filled her mind and body, and her arms responded to the movements she used on stage as a young ballerina.

When conversing with people became hard as confusion in her brain could not identify who they were, the music still found a crack where old memories could sneak into the brain again. Even though she was wheelchair-bound, her arms found expression in the music. Expression stole up into her face, reflecting her face as she danced in her youth.

CHANGES IN MODERATE (STAGE 5) DEMENTIA

This stage can last from one to five years. The average length is estimated to be around one and a half years. However, we must remember that every individual will progress at their own pace and will show some or all of the symptoms of this stage.

Your loved one may find it difficult to decide what to wear, so what they wore yesterday seems to be a good choice. The problem is that what they wore yesterday may have been worn for the previous X amount of days. They have lost the concept of cleanliness in their clothes. They take the clothes off, set them aside, and pick them up again the next day. They have also lost the concept of hot and cold days. So, on a cold day, they may be found in minimal clothing, and on a hot day, the jerseys may come out. The easiest way out of this is for you to grab their clothes as they come off and set out the clean set of clothing for tomorrow.

They may also need to be encouraged to bathe or take a shower, as this is no longer a priority in their lives. Zips and buttons could become difficult for them to handle, so pull-on tops and bottoms need to be considered.

You, as the caregiver, will need to step up your involvement in their lives. They will need help with cooking, paying bills, and dressing. As they battle to think logically, they will be depending on you for many decision-based things. You need to stay alert to any signs that your loved one may be struggling. When you see that they need help, keep a cool frame of mind as you step in. Don't just take over. Ask if they would like you to help them. Then, assist them and be ready to take over when the task gets too complicated for them.

Their memory will not be reliable, and they may forget who you are. They will probably not remember their address or phone number. This is concerning if they manage to slip out and do a walkabout. If they get lost, they will not be able to get back home by themselves or without the help of the police or helpful strangers. If you are worried about them getting lost, it might be an idea to stitch their details in their clothing. However, it is also time to check how secure their home is. No one wants to lock their loved ones inside all the time, but when they go out, they should be accompanied by someone responsible at all times. However, there is the possibility that the carer might be distracted long enough for the loved one to wander off. So better safe than sorry.

You will find them looking for words to express themselves more frequently than before. In this stage, an outgoing person may seem to undergo a change of personality, but it could simply be that they no longer have the confidence to express themselves in company. They may also become confused if too many people are conversing at once. This could also make them pull in and become uncommunicative. They don't need criticism or cajoling. What they do need is to feel that you are supportive of them no matter what.

DEMENTIA STAGE 5: MODERATELY SEVERE COGNITIVE DECLINE

Because of the severe decline in logic, reasoning, and memory, this is a tricky stage for the caregiver. It requires patience and love. You will hear the same story maybe three or four times during a session. You just have to smile and nod and ask the same questions that you did five minutes ago. You will be asked the same questions over and over again. It doesn't help you or the loved one to try to remind them that you have already answered the questions before, maybe many times. So, how can you deal with this? You will have to bite your tongue and distract them. If they like music, suggest you listen to some music. If they like to paint or draw, get those paints, paper, and pencils out and get them busy. If they enjoy cooking and a kitchen is available, get in there and make a bunch of tasty treats.

Don't be alarmed if they suddenly get tired of the distraction and snap at you or become angry or aggressive. It is not your loved one responding but the disease.

You will need to help them with going to the toilet, so you need to get over any hang-ups you may have. They will not be able to wipe their own bottom. Essentially, in many ways, you will have a feisty toddler on your hands.

Early on in the disease, you could have taken notes about how they would want to be treated during these late stages. If this didn't happen, your loved one is now not capable of thinking of solutions. Your best bet is to get help from organizations or fellow caregivers on how to deal with this stage.

Your confusion of how to proceed is nothing like the confusion that they will often feel. They will often be disorientated in a place that they formally knew. This will leave them confused, and they will need you to be calm and reassuring.

As dusk settles in, they could become restless, confused, and objectionable. This is a stage known as *sundowning*. You, as a carer, need to be the calming influence in their life.

This is a time when you will need patience and understanding as your loved one looks to you for stability in this frighteningly changing world.

COGNITIVE CHANGES IN MODERATELY SEVERE (STAGE 6) DEMENTIA

After an average of one and a half years, your loved one will move into stage 6 dementia. Some aspects of stage 6 will have started to evolve in stage 5 but will become more intense in this stage. It almost becomes an impossibility for you to handle this stage by yourself. You may have done well up to now, but you need to bring in relief staff at this point. Some aspects that will worsen are:

- Memory loss will become more evident. They will immediately forget previous events almost as they happen. Close family members must not be surprised if they are not recognized. Places that they have visited in the past will not be recognized or be confused. They may think that their child is their mother or their cousin is their father.
- Your loved one will have increasing difficulty in communicating with you. They will not find the words to express themselves, and they could become easily frustrated if you do not know that the word (for example) door actually means that they want food. Words become meaningless to them. You will need to become more aware of their nonverbal communication.
- Personality and mood changes will become more evident as your loved one grapples with who you and other people are in their life. They could become more easily frustrated at not being understood.

- Their delusions and hallucinations will increase. They may be convinced that they have to get ready for work.
- They will need more help with intimate things like going to the toilet, bathing, and dressing. Their bladder control could worsen.
- The will to wander will become stronger, and you will have to be extremely vigilant as, if left to their own devices, they will become lost and vulnerable to the criminal element in the vicinity.
- They will become tired during the day and will want to sleep, which will disrupt their sleep at night.
- Their taste in food may change, and something that they previously loved to eat may be refused.

Your patience will be tested. Music will often help your loved one relax and may even bring up hidden memories. Reading to them will also help, but please remember that tomorrow, they will have no recollection of what was read today.

W.G.'s Story

W.G. relates that he was a student when his mother was diagnosed with dementia. As he was away during term time, it was easy for him to see the changes in his mom's condition when he came home for the holidays. As his mom entered the late stages of dementia, it became impossible to keep her at home as he and his brother were studying away from home and his dad was working.

It gave them peace of mind that she was safe during the times when no one was available to care for her. His father described the disease as gradual bereavement, which just about sums it up—his loved one gradually retreats from you until they slip away.

The last years were very difficult as she lost the sense of communicating, and they could seldom get more from her other than a grunt.

The impact of the disease chewed away at W.G., and his studying took a toll, with him failing some courses. He also became reclusive, but when his thoughts got the better of him, he resorted to going out drinking while never letting on to his mates about his mom's condition. His advice to everyone going through this is to talk about it and talk to friends, family, or counselors. Do not bottle it up because it could cause you to wreck your own life. Fortunately, W.G. came to his senses and got the help he needed, as well as opening up to his friends.

E and B's Story

E was in his last year in elementary school when his dad, B, was diagnosed with dementia. When he transferred to middle school, he was scared to invite friends home in case they judged him badly because of his father, as he could never be sure what state his dad would be in when he got home from school. E noticed that his dad would smile, even when other forms of communication stopped, and he would catch a glimpse of the father he wished to remember.

B was a musician, and they found that playing music soothed him. On a good day, even though talking was no longer possible, he could play the piano.

EMOTIONAL AND BEHAVIORAL ASPECTS

As dementia progresses, your loved one's agitation will increase. There are many factors which can lead to increased agitation, some being as follows:

- Any change in the environment. This may be new drapes, new furniture, or a change in where they live. You might have moved them to a care facility and they feel strange.
- The caregiver may be a new person, and they may have difficulty relating to them.
- They may have developed a new strange fear that is making them agitated.
- They may just be hungry or thirsty and not be able to communicate properly.

Remember that dementia is a disease of the brain, and there is no real forecasting of which part of the brain will be affected next. They need to be reassured that everything is safe and you are a constant.

Use all the tricks that you have built up over the years of caring to find the trigger that will calm them down. This trigger might be music, reading to them, getting them up and active using yoga, or just a simple walk in a garden.

As they may not be able to communicate that they are sore, always bear this in mind when calming them down. Take note of any winces as you touch them, as this may help you isolate pain should any exist.

Their environment may be over-stimulating, and there may be too much going on, which is confusing to them. Try to keep every-thing simple like:

- using simple language
- dealing with one thing at a time
- be understanding as you listen to them trying to communicate their problems

Remember to make a note of anything new in their behavior so that you can report on it during their next visit.

Another aspect that may develop during this stage is aggression and anger. The causes will be similar to what causes agitation. In a way, anger and aggression is like agitation on steroids. This means that you could use similar techniques to help your loved one during this phase.

You will be called on to help your loved one with eating, supervising dressing, bathing, and toilet visits. You may have to consider adult incontinence wear as your loved one may be confused as to signals that they need the toilet.

E and N

The problem with dementia is that grieving starts while the person is still with you. You repeatedly grieve over the bits of them that have been lost. You grieve for the person that they were. You grieve for the fact that they won't see or recognize their grandchildren. And then you grieve when the disease has taken them away completely.

The emotional impact of dealing with a person with dementia continues for months after their death. E speaks about her mother N.

While her mother was alive, there were things to do and things to see to. Caring for her while she was living with E was easy as the family mucked in and helped as much as they could. When N had to be transferred to a care facility, the emotions of having to make that decision rested solely with the immediate family, and she was the only person in her immediate family. It was up to her to find a suitable place; up to her to move her mother; up to her to be the punch bag when her mother reacted to the move; and also up to her to visit each day, preferably at different times, in order to maintain contact with her disappearing mom.

After her mother's death, she handled all the end-of-life issues, and once that was taken care of, she thought she could begin piecing her life together at last. This was when she found that she wasn't coping with daily life. She started having panic attacks where she wanted to just hide from reality. A counselor explained that this was grieving and that she had to allow herself time to grieve.

She found that journaling and yoga helped her when she felt she could no longer cope.

Tips to Deal With the Three As

Anger, Aggression, and Anxiety make up the three As that you might encounter while caring for your loved one. In all situations, it is important to remain as calm as possible. If the carer gets over excited, this will be picked up by your loved one and will probably make their reactions extreme. Other things to consider are:

- Remember that you are not alone. There is always someone at the end of a telephone call. It may be a relative, a friend, or a professional. Do not try to deal with things by yourself. Remember that old adage: A problem shared is a problem halved.
- If you need a break, make sure you take it before it takes you out. Engage the help of friends and relatives to step in when you need a few hours for yourself. If you need more time, think of getting your loved one into a care situation for a few days or a week or so. There will usually be a respite home in fairly close proximity. This break will also

help you step away from the problem, and you will be able to see your solutions with a clearer focus.

- During the three As, your loved one may have unimaginable strength. Don't try to restrain them by yourself. Make sure you have a contact that can get to you quickly in the case of an emergency. A good neighbor is the ideal situation. Reassure them that they will only be called on in an emergency.
- Most situations can be diffused early if you keep a sense of humor. If that doesn't work, try to distract them.

PHYSICAL CHANGES AND CARE NEEDS

As your loved one enters the final two stages of dementia, things will start to change.

- They will no longer be able to do simple tasks like feeding themselves.
- They will either be bedridden or will need help getting around.
- Swallowing food could be a challenge, and the carer may have to resort to a liquid diet or even feed them via a tube.
- There will be confusion between day and night, and they will probably not get a full night's sleep. This will be an impossible situation for a carer operating alone, and a night nurse or outside carer will have to be considered.
- The confusion between day and night could lead to anxiety attacks or the need to wander.

All of the above places an incredible burden on the carer both physically and mentally. If your loved one is bedridden, you will have to learn how to do bed baths, attend to bed sores, and move your loved one so that the physical impact on yourself is minimized.

PALLIATIVE CARE AND PAIN MANAGEMENT

Palliative care is offered to people living with a serious health issue. The family of the patient is helped to tend to the patient and is also educated in ways to help the patient during this stressful time. During palliative care, the patient is kept as free from pain as possible. The symptoms of terminal illnesses are treated in a way that makes the patient as comfortable as possible during this transition to the end-of-life phase.

Palliative care is offered to anyone who needs comfort, support, and pain management while handling severe health issues. It could also be used in end-of-life situations. It is available to any patient. All that is needed is one doctor's recommendation.

Palliative care follows the advice of Dame Cicely Saunders (n.d.) (nurse, physician writer, and founder of the modern-day hospice movement): "You matter because you are you, and you matter to the end of your life. We will do all we can not only to help you die peacefully but also to live until you die."

CREATING A SAFE AND SUPPORTIVE ENVIRONMENT

If you decide to keep your loved one at home with you for as long as possible, certain modifications will need to be made. One of the important things is to label everything. The door to their bedroom, the toilet door, and all other doors. Utensil holders should be named as well. Kitchen appliances need identifying labels. It is important to follow the idiom "A place for everything and everything in its place" if you label appliances. A misplaced appliance could be interpreted incorrectly. For example, placing the toaster where the kettle belongs will confuse your loved one as their logical brain is dying. Some other aspects are:

- Furnishings and accessories should be kept as plain as possible. Jazzy patterns will confuse your loved one.
- Doors leading outside should be kept locked, and keys stored far away.
- Trip hazards, like loose carpets, need to be attended to. Your loved one, particularly if they are suffering from Parkinson's disease, will shuffle along the floor rather than walk. Check on loose electrical cords as well.
- Grab bars in the bathroom and toilet are essential.
- You need to ensure that there is good lighting in the home. A night light in your loved one's room will be calming to them.

Chat with your health professional about other safety measures. They may be able to give you a contact who can assess your home for other changes that might be needed.

Remember that your loved one's judgment and logic will be faulty. They may also have problems with depth perception as well as other visual problems.

CAREGIVER SELF-CARE AND EMOTIONAL WELL-BEING

If you need to take care of your loved one, your own self-care is your number one priority. You cannot afford to get caregiver burnout. Your job with your loved one is a full-time occupation, but so is caring for your other family and maybe even trying to keep up with the demands of a career. The stress of keeping all these balls in the air could lead to depression, sleep issues, and heart problems, and the immune system could weaken. So, your self-care has an impact on how you can best care for your loved one.

If you find yourself dealing with any of the following problems, you need to get help for yourself:

- being over-anxious about how you are coping
- living with a short fuse where you are liable to overreact to situations
- being tired all the time
- finding that your attention span is shortened and you get distracted easily

If you find you are suffering from any one of these symptoms, speak to your medical advisor or other health care professional. It might mean putting your loved one in a respite home for a couple of weeks until you can cope again.

Effective Self-Care Strategies

You must establish what you can do for your loved one, but it is more important to establish what you can do to keep yourself in tip-top shape. There are basically five areas to look at when considering self-care:

- Physical self-care—are you...
  - getting enough sleep?
  - getting enough exercise?
  - eating correctly?
- Emotional self-care—do you...
  - have someone who can support you emotionally?

- have strategies to help you cope?
- Spiritual self-care—do you...
  - have a spiritual outlet?
  - feel yourself blessed?
  - give yourself time to listen to the answers when you question yourself?
- Mental self-care—do you...
  - spend time doing something you enjoy?

The above three subsections will also provide you with sources you can apply for mental self-care.

- Emotional self-care—do you...
  - give yourself time to relax?

Again, all the subsections above will give you emotional support.

You may need to continually remind yourself that you are part of a team. You are not alone on this caregiving trip. It is also important that you don't take guilt along with you. Forget about beating yourself up with statements like:

- I should have done that differently.
- I should not have lost my temper.
- I should have been more careful.

Remember that the person you are caring for will have forgotten the situation in the next half hour.

COPING WITH GRIEF AND LOSS

Death comes to all of us, so theoretically, we all know how to handle grief, but the grief of death from dementia is something different. Some say that the last stages of dementia are like a living death. The family knows the outcome but just does not know when it will hit. As their loved one loses a grip on their faculties, there is grief, and the grief intensifies as each faculty disappears. The family starts to live in anticipatory grief as they know what lies before them but do not know how long their anticipatory grief will last.

Karen Wilder, who was her husband's (Gene Wilder) primary caregiver until he died in 2016, sums this up nicely:

"The hardest part was losing him every minute of every day. I could see him receding, and that made me sick to my stomach," Karen says. "I held it in. I would smile and try to make things happy for him. But I was watching him disappear" (ALZ Magazine, 2020).

Karen chose to deal with her grief at losing him by becoming an advocate for helping others in a similar situation. She uses scenes from his movies to help people understand the immensity of the disease.

The best advice to any caregiver will be to live in the moment. Appreciate the small things that give you a glimpse of the person who your loved one was. Do not look forward and do not look back; appreciate and live now. Karen is grateful that his sense of humor did not abandon him during his struggle with the disease.

Coping With Grief

When your loved one dies, you suddenly find yourself with so much time on your hands. As you start to go through their things, memories will crop up. Treasure those memories.

No time span is correct for the grieving process. Take all the time you need. You have let a part of yourself go, and you need time to adjust to life without your loved one. Death is so final. Your loved one will never return, and you need to be able to deal with it in your own way and in your own time. No one can dictate how long it should take. In some religions, there is an official mourning period, but you need not stick to that if it doesn't suit you. Just be aware that your life has continued, and you need to adjust to life without your loved one.

Jamie Anderson has a memorable quote on grief. "Grief, I've learned, is really just love. It's all the love you want to give, but cannot. All that unspent love gathers up in the corners of your eyes, the lump in your throat, and in that hollow part of your chest. Grief is just love with no place to go" (n.d.).

Five Stages of Grief

In order to help you understand grief and that what you are feeling is a legitimate emotion, there are five stages that a person normally goes through during grieving.

- **Denial:** This is your first reaction. It cannot be true.
- **Anger:** This can be directed at yourself, your deity, or the person who has left you.
- **Bargaining:** You try to make deals with yourself, others, or your deity.
- **Acceptance:** At this point, you accept that there is going to be a hole in your life that nobody can fill, but you are prepared to go out into the world again, and your memories of the person become treasure troves.

If, at any point in your grieving process, you feel you need help, there are support groups. These can also be found on social media. You could also seek professional help.

SEGUE

Chapter 1 seems to have thrown you in the deep end, but I hope it has been helpful. In the next chapter, we will look at person-centered care and how you can manage your loved one in a caring manner that is suited to both of you.

CHAPTER TWO

PROVIDING PERSON-CENTERED CARE

If you learn to listen for clues as to how I feel instead of what I say, you will be able to understand me much better.

— MARA BOTONIS

I f you have chosen to be the principal caregiver for your loved one, you will be faced with many tough decisions along the way. As your loved one enters the final stages of this disease, you will need to decide if they would be better off with outside care, like palliative care or hospice care, or if they would be better off staying with you. Whatever you decide, whether by yourself or in consultation with other family members, will be the correct choice for your unique situation.

If you have chosen to care for your loved one, you will have chosen to center your care on your loved one's abilities, interests, and comfort. Many carers choose that path because they want their loved ones to be comfortable in their own space. If you choose this route, you need to keep in mind that you will need help, if not now, then eventually. Intimate issues are often a reason why a carer fails or comes close to failing, as the loss of dignity of their loved ones plays on the carer's mind.

You also need to consider the very real prospect of carer burnout. If you face burnout, your loved one will not get the care they need. Get help sooner or later. You will also need to be taught how to lift a person who is bed-bound.

B and J

B has taken care of her husband, J, since his diagnosis. They met when they were 14 years old and were married at 21 years of age. She cherishes the time that she gets to spend with J and has done whatever is necessary to discover how to make these last years of their marriage as meaningful as the previous years have been.

She says that finding people in a similar position has been a lifeline and encourages other carers to join associations where they can get whatever help they need. She urges others to live each day to the fullest. Each day will bring fresh challenges, but all you can do is do your best.

UNDERSTANDING PERSON-CENTERED CARE

The Gerontologist has an excellent definition of Person-Centered care "Person-centered care is a philosophy of care built around the needs of the individual and contingent upon knowing the person through an interpersonal relationship" (Fazio et al., 2018).

Hospitals are normally dictated by the clock: Shifts start and end on the clock, and medication and baths are done on the clock. With person-centered care, the carer and other staff work with your loved one to adjust everything to suit your loved one. Timing becomes flexible, and activities are brought in to suit the mood and abilities of your loved one. These may, and probably will, differ from day to day. The caregiver focus should be on what they need to do to ensure their loved one's comfort. It should be immaterial when things are done or how things are done. Your loved one's intrinsic self can still be found even far into the late stages of dementia. You, as a carer, need to encourage visitors to treat your loved one as they have been treating them before the disease took them over. This is more likely to get a positive response from your loved one during those visits.

The Concept of Person-Centered Care

This concept has several core principles:

- **Comfort:** If you could get into the mind of a person with dementia, you would understand that they are confused and feel as if they were not in control of their lives. Use words of comfort together with actions. Reassure your loved one. That all you wish for is for them to feel comfortable in their situation. Some dementia sufferers find comfort in dolls; they can rock them and soothe them, and this somehow manages to soothe the person as well.
- **Attachment:** Life can sometimes be very confusing for a dementia sufferer. If they have to be moved because you find that you are struggling with full-time care, they will take a while to settle into strange surroundings. It will be beneficial to pack some familiar items for them. Some carer facilities allow them to bring their own furniture with them. If they can't have their own familiar furniture, then pack their favorite blankets and other personal items.
- **Inclusion:** They are still there, in a different way, perhaps, but they need to be acknowledged. Decision-making will

be difficult, but offering them two options will make it easier. If you say, "What would you like to do?" your loved one may find it hard to remember all the things that they loved doing, but if you change that to "Would you like to paint or listen to music?" The choice and decision will be easier.

- **Occupation:** Make sure your loved one does not sit for hours on end staring at a blank wall. Ensure that you have ample distractions at your fingertips. Keep a photograph album or scrapbook close at hand. A delve into their personal history will also keep your loved one focused. Play music, dance, or sing. Nearly everyone can associate with music. Read to them from a book, newspaper, or magazine. Go for a walk. Play a favorite game. All these activities can make sure that your loved one is not left for hours with no stimulation. Be sure to try different activities when you notice your loved one losing interest.

- **Identity:** Always remember that they have an identity. Although the disease may have robbed them of many things, they will still have their likes and dislikes.
  - ○ Don de Vlaming, an Alzheimer sufferer, enjoys the company that he finds in his dementia support group. He says that while he enjoys time with his friends and family, they have preconceived ideas about him. His contacts at the support group did not know him prior to his time in the group, so everyone listens to what is being said. No one is judgmental. Everyone respects each other. He feels that those who do not suffer from dementia do not fully understand the world that dementia sufferers inhabit (Alzheimer Society Manitoba, 2012).

BENEFITS OF PERSON-CENTERED CARE

A person with dementia can be relegated to the sidelines. Person-centered care aims to include the dementia patient in all things medical, social, and personal. In this, carers in a care facility need to work closely with family members to ensure that loved ones are settled in their new environment. If you still have your loved one at home, you are probably already following the tenets that will suit your loved one.

The policies in person-centered care include the following:

- Care for your loved one with respect.
- Respect their need for social exposure.
- Respect their preferences for activities that suit their personalities.
- Ensure that their dignity remains intact.
- Follow a course of treatment that protects their dignity and sits well with their beliefs and needs.
- Build a partnership with your loved one to work together within their abilities.

The advantages of person-centered care (also called patient-centered care) are:

- Your loved one feels more in control of their life.
- They will meet others in a similar situation to themselves.
- Their daytime activities will be enjoyed more if you heed their input and personalities.
- Intimate care will be less threatening.
- They will feel more useful when they have a say in their daily life.

Person-centered care will need a flexible framework. While this is not the easiest thing to comply with in a hospital-like setting, it is not impossible. For this to succeed, the staff need to be open-minded and also need to work with the person's family and other loved ones. A deeper bond between the carer, institution, and patient will be forged.

THE ROYAL MELBOURNE HOSPITAL CASE STUDY

When Lola's daughter complained about the quality of care that her mother had received, instead of just sweeping the complaint under the mat, the hospital decided to develop a more person-centered approach and film it with Lola and her family. The resultant movie, *Lola's Story*, illustrates the road the hospital took. Lola's daughter was an experienced aged care professional and was happy to help with the development of more patient-orientated care.

Lola's story was followed by another movie dealing with another patient, *Florence's Story*. These two movies are used to help with staff training sessions.

IMPLEMENTING PERSON-CENTERED CARE PRACTICES

Person-centered care has to take into account that each person has their own character, their own likes and dislikes, and their own preferences. In other words, people cannot be treated in a one-size-fits-all-all way.

Person-centered care takes all of the above into account, and the staff is trained to put the person first and the institution second. This is particularly important when dealing with dementia patients. Each patient is different and can have a say in how they wish to be treated, both medically, spiritually, and personally.

Staff in hospitals and other institutions will have to attend training sessions as this way of dealing with patients does not fully align with the way they have been working for many years, so the change from institution-centered care to person-centered care may be met with a bit of opposition. Yes, it may be more time-consuming, but the staff will be dealing with happier people.

Staff will also be building a better relationship with their charges. People with late-stage dementia can be resistant to new people, but if you take an interest in who they are and what they like, your course of treatment will become easier.

If you take the time to talk to your patients and really listen to them, you will gain their respect, and they will be more willing to go along with you. Question them, look at their photograph albums or scrapbooks. Become an empathetic listener. They will be more willing to meet you halfway and let you know what they want and if they want their treatment to progress.

Understand that they will be battling with the correct words to make their feelings known. This could lead to them withdrawing. Do whatever it takes to break those barriers to communication. Maybe they won't know how to tell you that they are hungry, so use words and actions to help identify their problem.

- Talk slowly and clearly, but never talk down to them.
- Keep your tone of voice calm and quiet, and use simple vocabulary.
- Don't present them with more than one idea or two choices. More will confuse them.
- Smile when you see them and rejoice when they smile back at you.
- Keep the surroundings uncluttered and quiet; a blaring TV can be upsetting to a person with dementia.

- Keep still while communicating. If you are buzzing around the room, tidying up, or pulling the bed straight, their attention will move to your actions, as words are much harder to understand.
- Coerce rather than issue orders.
- Don't ask them to remember previous events, but encourage them to talk about any memories they may have. A photo album or scrapbook will help jolt their memory. What happened yesterday will be forgotten as short-term memory cannot be retained for long. When we do not have dementia, things that are in the short-term memory get moved to a more retentive part of the brain. This is disrupted in dementia.
- Encourage them to keep up their interests, even if that means simply sticking Christmas cards into a scrapbook.
- They can hear and process things that are said in front of them. Do not demean them or talk about their condition as if they are not even in the room.

You, the carer, will have to explore many ways to communicate as the dementia progresses.

Therapies You Can Explore

Some therapies that have proved to be helpful when dealing with dementia sufferers are:

- music
- movement
- enter their world rather than trying to get them to live in your world
- help them build up their own personal history with photos and cards in a scrapbook

INDIVIDUALIZED CARE PLANS AND DECISION-MAKING

Creating individualized care plans allows healthcare providers to tailor treatment strategies to meet the unique needs of each patient. Collaborative decision-making ensures that patients are actively involved in their treatment options, enhancing their overall experience and satisfaction.

Individualized care plans form an integral part of personal-centered care services. It is important that patients know that they can control their care package. Any decisions taken must involve the patient, but family carers should also be part of the plan. The family carer has gone through the ropes and knows their loved one's likes and dislikes.

The hospital or institution's staff must be prepared to listen to all the suggestions in order to build up a unique care package. They must ensure that the person's feelings are validated and care will be offered according to the person's experiences. Hobbies will also be taken into consideration. All of this will lead to a more cooperative and happier person.

What to Include

There are a few things that need to be included in generating a person-centered care package:

- Make the environment pleasant. This could include personal items, playing music that talks to the person, and greeting them with a smile. A smile is infectious. It is hard to greet a smile with a somber or sullen expression. The very act of smiling will lighten the person's mood, making interaction pleasant.

- Take into consideration that while short-term memory is not reliable, the person in front of you has memories and life achievements, so where possible, display trophies, medals, and so on.
- Interact in a personal rather than a professional manner.

Things That Will Improve

When dealing with a dementia patient, aggression is often not far away. Building up an individualized care package will diminish the incidences of aggression.

There will be an improvement in:

- the person's confidence
- medication needs
- stress triggers

CREATING A COMFORTING AND SUPPORTIVE ENVIRONMENT

As carers, we need to provide an environment that will help our loved ones relax and be as much themselves as possible. We can do this by using the following techniques:

- Make sure that the lighting is comfortable, not too bright, which can be disconcerting, and not so dim that reading will be affected.
- If you are redecorating, colors should be calming and muted. That startling orange wall that you love needs to go.
- Memories scattered around the room will help your reminiscing sessions.

- Favorite accessories like blankets, books, and other trinkets that can help your loved one settle.
- Music that is restful or favorite music selections will also help your loved one relax in the setting.
- Make sure that the bathroom has grab handles and a note on the door indicating (preferably in pictures and words) the purpose of the room.

A supportive environment involves you, the carer, in a meaningful way.

- Always greet them with a smile.
- When communicating, use words, gestures, and facial expressions, and remember to talk slowly.
- Listen to your loved one with your whole attention so that you can pick up threads to explore more fully.
- Be ready to soothe away their concerns about where they are.

PROMOTING AUTONOMY AND DECISION-MAKING

This is what person-centered care is all about. You want your loved one to

- make decisions as to what activities they want to engage in. Yesterday, it may have been dance, but today, maybe they want you to read to them. Remember not to ask open questions like "What would you like to do today?" Instead, offer two choices so your question will become, "Do you want to paint or dance today?" Be prepared to have two other choices in case they don't want to do either, but don't bombard them with many choices, as that is confusing.

- perform the activity to the best of their ability. Praise is always welcome, but make sure your tone is not condescending. Your loved one is not a child and will pick up on the tone.

These considerations will help your loved one feel in control. It will enhance the sense of dignity and self. Remember to make sure that all activities are done in a safe environment, paying attention to the safety of your loved one.

If you ever have to take over the decision-making, make sure that you keep your loved one's dignity and rights. If your loved one finds decision-making difficult today, tomorrow may be a better day for them, so if the decision is not vitally important, leave it for another day. You may also need to consider other family members or other carers, so be sure to get their opinions before making an irreversible decision.

A study in the British Medical Journal concluded that shared decision-making in persons with dementia is possible. The experiment looked at whether or not the patient wanted to participate in a daycare program. It stressed that a patient's viewpoint may change depending on whether or not they had previously experienced daycare. The most positive results of the experiment endorsed that all parties should be able to have their input. If your loved one is battling to accept new ideas or activities, try to convince them that a decision cannot be made until they have tried the new activity. Once they have tried it, they will be able to decide if it is right for them (Groen-van de Ven et al., 2017).

SEGUE

Person-centered care is definitely the way to go for dementia patients. No two cases are alike. They will have several similar conditions and symptoms, but their innate personality will sway those symptoms and conditions so that they are presented slightly differently from other sufferers. No medical care should be a one-size-fits-all system, but it is great that dementia sufferers are paving the way for other conditions to be cared for in ways that are unique to the patient.

The next chapter is going to be looking at communication and sometimes the lack thereof. We will consider different methods of communicating with our loved ones. We will also discover how to help our loved ones when communication has become limited.

CHAPTER THREE

COMMUNICATION TECHNIQUES AND STRATEGIES

We believe communicating effectively with someone with Alzheimer's is not just about using language, it is connecting through their senses such as touch, visual cues and sound.

— PETER ROSS

As the dementia progresses, there will be a marked deterioration in the person's ability to participate in conversation. They will have difficulty finding the right words and following the logistics of a conversation.

As the late stages of dementia progress, the following will be noted:

- Your loved one will be at more of a loss for words as words disappear into the damaged area of their brain.
- The absence of logic means that they will have a problem following conversations, even when you remember to speak slowly to them.

- As word memory becomes faint, they will substitute meaningless words into their conversations in an attempt to be understood.

This chapter will help you, the carer, communicate with your loved one. Various strategies will be discussed.

UNDERSTANDING COMMUNICATION CHANGES IN LATE-STAGE DEMENTIA

The following are general observations, as every case of dementia has its own shortfalls:

Changes in Verbal Communication

It is very frustrating when you can't find the right word to express a thought. Late-stage dementia patients lose their ability to communicate as words don't come easy, and they battle to follow conversations. They will also have problems stringing words together to form a coherent sentence. This results in them withdrawing from social events even with people who are closely related.

As a carer, before you make any decision that your loved one has entered the non-communication cycle of the disease, you need to check two things:

- **Hearing:** Are they battling to hear? Is it an ear wax problem? A doctor could easily sort that one out. If they still do not hear well, they may have started lip reading to facilitate their failing sense. A quick test is to talk to them while concealing your lips behind a newspaper, menu, or even just by dropping your head. If they can't tell what you are saying, it may be time to consider hearing aids.

- **Sight:** They may need new spectacles. This could upset their balance. Eyes should be tested at least every two years.

We are all different, so the way that your loved one's dementia proceeds will not be identical to anyone else. As discussed earlier, there are various reasons why their ability to communicate deteriorates.

- Vocabulary decreases as the brain damage spreads. This makes having a reasonable conversation difficult. There will be many stops as your loved one tries to get the word to express his thoughts. They will often say a word that has little or no validity in the present conversation.
- Using an incorrect word starts to spread from general conversation to other aspects of their life. They will soon lose vocabulary that describes basic ideas like "I am hungry." or "I am tired." They may substitute words that enable you to decrypt their thoughts, like they may say "Ham" or "Blanket." But most of the time, the words may appear nonsensical. This means you have to employ other means to decipher what they mean.
- When you talk to your loved one, you need to keep your sentences short and speak clearly. They may only hear a portion of what you say, and that will not make any sense. This is because their brain damage does not allow them to concentrate fully on what has been said and the words may appear meaningless. Remember that their vocabulary is decreasing, which means their words as well as yours.
- Because the brain controls everything we do, your loved one may start to battle to use their hands and legs. Writing

becomes difficult as their fingers may not be able to grasp a pen or a pencil with enough pressure to write.

- Reading is also a problem as the patterns that letters make on a page may not be transferred to meaningful words. The sentences may be too long and include too many thoughts to follow.
- They may interrupt conversations taking place around them. This would be seen as being rude to anyone not suffering from dementia. But the niceties of polite conversation are lost on them. If they have a thought, they need to get it out there, and then, in a couple of minutes, they will have forgotten it.
- Their emotions may get the better of them. This could also be because they have forgotten the words to express their emotions. This could lead to an outbreak similar to a tantrum of a two-year-old.

All of this means you need to discover new ways to interact with your loved one.

NONVERBAL COMMUNICATION AND BODY LANGUAGE

When you are trying to build up a conversation with a person who is suffering from dementia, you need to watch:

- **Body language:** This is important as your loved one will be watching you to help them understand what you are trying to say. Keep your responses kind and positive. A sigh or tense lips are not positive body language signs, and while your loved one may not understand why you are reacting like that, they will know that you are venting disapproval. A smile can do wonders. You need to watch your loved one's body language as well. You may catch them looking longingly at someone who is eating or drinking near them. Pick up on this and ask if they are hungry. You can accompany this by pretending to put food in your mouth. In this way, they will understand the action even if the words are meaningless. If they want to sleep, you may notice a general relaxing of the body as it sinks into itself, or maybe their eyes are heavy, or they are yawning. Body language signs are usually present and can be used to add meaning to your verbal content.

- **Physical touch:** If it is acceptable to your loved one, you can also use touch to help get your point across. A touch on the arm, an arm around their shoulders, or just holding hands may help them stay calm as you are talking. In a calm state, they will be able to understand more of what you are saying.

- **Your voice:** Keep the tone of your voice friendly and calm when you address your loved one. Try not to let exasperation take over. There will probably be many times that you will be adversely affected by their situation. If you keep your tone calm, it will help calm you down as well. They will respond well to a calm tone.

- **Your words:** As said before, simple words and sentences are best, and when coupled with your calm voice and actions, you will find that understanding once again develops between you. You will need to wait a bit longer after speaking to allow them to assimilate and act on your words.

Always try to keep them in a conversation. Don't talk over them, and don't give your attention to someone else in the conversation to the exclusion of them.

T.H.

T.H.'s mother is virtually catatonic. She has suffered from dementia for at least ten years. When she was younger and working, she used a typewriter a lot and would often sit watching TV while her fingers played a silent tune in her lap. One of his visits left him feeling much more positive about his mom's condition. They were sitting together. He was chatting to her while holding her hand, and soon, there was that old familiar habit of fingers moving on a keyboard. This left him feeling that maybe, in her mind, she was still capable of coherent thought and used her fingers to type out her message.

EMOTIONAL AND SENSORY COMMUNICATION

If you want to carry on a conversation with a dementia patient, make sure that there are no distracting noises like a blaring TV or a noisy, crowded room. The less distraction, the easier it will be to chat with your loved one.

Your loved one will often be confused, which will lead to anxiety. They will cope best in an environment that has muted tones and muted sounds. Keep the décor simple. Display mementos that are meaningful to your loved one.

Dementia robs the person of the ability to communicate in the conventional method, but the emotional part of the brain is still very active. This means that you will have to adapt to their method of communicating because they can't relearn your methods of communicating.

Sounds, scents, tastes, and textures evoke memories in all of us. Using items that stimulate these memories will help keep your loved one calm. Sensory communication with dementia sufferers is gaining popularity, and the world around us offers many things that can be used in sensory therapy.

- You can collect samples of different types of sand, from beach sand to garden sand and all textures in between. Flowers and leaves can be felt, rubbed, smelt, and admired, thus engaging, feel, smell, touch, and sight.
- You can collect different sounds: a river flowing, whale noises, bells, music, and bird sounds can evoke memories that can stimulate sensory delight.
- When throwing out clothing or cloths, collect them together and use them for stimulating touch. Get a selection of rough and soft. Use knitted garments to introduce a different feel. Try to have different colors represented.
- Collect a group of items and have a blind taste session. If verbalizing their answers is difficult, give them word clues like "Is it sour?" "Is it sweet?" and so on. You can use cinnamon, lemon, sugar, salt, pepper, and many more.

You want to make your leisure time together pleasant and meaningful. I have already mentioned the idea of using a photograph album or a scrapbook to encourage communication as well. All the above activities will often stimulate long-forgotten memories, taking the activity on a broader journey. The activities will also help your loved one:

- feel safe
- relax
- enjoy remembered times again
- moods
- gain a sense of well-being

Music

Most people respond well to music. It opens up a feel-good space in the brain, particularly with dementia sufferers. This could help open up communication between the carer and the patient as it often helps settle and calm the patient. If you play music to your loved one, It should help bring a little clarity to a clouded brain. This could open the door to communicating in a meaningful way. It can bring laughter back to their lives, even if for only a short time.

If you play songs from their youth, they may surprise you by singing along. They may even be moved to dance.

At the end-of-life stage, music may settle them and help them relax. It is interesting to note that of all the senses, hearing remains the longest.

Music will also help get your loved one to move. Their dancing may not be "Dancing With the Stars" style, but they will certainly move better when you inspire them with music.

Dolls

Surprisingly, many dementia patients (both male and female) respond to holding and nursing dolls. While they cannot be trusted to look after a live baby, a doll seems to bring comfort and a sense of responsibility to dementia sufferers. You could use a doll to help discover where they are hurting.

It has been observed that dementia patients smile more, and challenging behaviors decrease. When your loved one is experiencing sundowning, a doll may bring calmness to them.

Some advocates against using dolls feel that it is demeaning to give a grown-up a doll to play with. As a caregiver, you have the ability to decide whether or not you want to explore this route.

Pets

Caring for pets is beyond the abilities of late-stage dementia patients, but it is a fact that the presence of pets can keep a dementia sufferer calm down during their bad periods.

Tom Stevens came up with a solution that helped his mom deal with the loss of a pet. Initially, he bought her toy dogs, but she did not like them. So, in 2017, his company created a dog robot, or Tombot, called Jennie. Jennie is a remarkable eight to ten-week-old Golden Labrador pup look alike. Jennie is a lap dog with many inbuilt features that imitate a real live dog. Jennie can bark, wag her tail, and respond to being petted. If the owner has not interacted with her for long, she goes to sleep, complete with a gentle snore.

Jennie works on a rechargeable battery, so in a way, she is the last word in plug-and-play pets.

EFFECTIVE COMMUNICATION STRATEGIES

Although these have been discussed before, a quick relook at these techniques may be helpful. When communicating with someone who has dementia, remember these few ideas to help you get the best out of your time with them.

- Keep all comments, explanations, and sentences short, and use simple language. Repeat if necessary, but be careful to keep your tone free from exasperation. Repeat as if this was the first time you were saying it.

- Don't bombard your loved one with many ideas at a time. Present one sentence, wait for them to hear, assess, and only then respond. Because of their vocabulary difficulties, they will not be capable of an immediate response.
- Agree with your loved one even if you know they are wrong. Turn it around by saying something like, "Sorry, I forgot you didn't like fish." even if fish has been their favorite food for as long as you remember. You are the responsible one in this relationship. You just need to go with what they think is right.
- Their logic has become unreliable, so reasoning, arguing, and reminding them will only frustrate both of you. They cannot remember what happened yesterday, so don't force the issue. For instance, if they saw a movie yesterday but today they complain that it has been so long since they saw a movie, just agree with words like, "Yes, I know. We must make sure we go soon."

With all these communication restrictions it's forgivable if you sometimes misstep. It's forgivable if your fuse gets short. Before you explode, make an excuse to get out of the room and cool down. Remember that they cannot help it; their memory fails them more each day, so if they blow up in your face, you cannot take this personally.

Active Listening and Validation

When you are chatting with your loved one, you need to ensure that you are actively listening to them. This is for a few reasons:

- With their incomplete grasp of necessary words, you may get the wrong idea if your attention has wandered.

- Your time with your loved one is precious; don't squander it on letting your brain wander into inconsequentials.
- If they are having a good day, you will find that conversing is easy and enjoyable if you lose yourself in the moment. Moments like this will become rare, so enjoy them by actively participating in the chat.
- You are chatting with an adult whose word usage has diminished but whose observation is probably still very good, and they will see if you are not actively participating.

When actively listening, there will be eye contact and changes of expression. You will nod or shake your head in response to their comments.

When you take your loved one's feelings and emotions into consideration, you are proving to them that you understand what they are going through and that you validate their feelings and situation. It is worse than useless to try to correct them or reason with them. Use your words, touch, or gestures to convey your understanding.

Visual Aids and Assistive Communication Tools

Pictures can be used to facilitate your communication. The use of scrapbooks and photograph albums has already been discussed. But how about pictures of emojis? Your loved one battles to find words to express their feelings. So, if you make a set of cards with definite emojis, you can show them a card, one at a time, and ask if that picture represents their feelings. You can take this concept further by finding pictures that will help them establish if they are hot, cold, hungry, tired, and so on.

"Coffee table" books are also a great way to pass the time. These big, colorful books with many pictures and limited text will enable you to spend many hours communicating with your loved one. There is a wide variety of these books: some are travel, some are geographic, some are of animals, and some are inspirational.

Utilizing Assistive Communication Tools

As technology improves, items are being developed to help people with dementia. We have already discussed the robot dog, but there are many more aids:

- Get a clock with a big clear face so that your loved one may be able to figure out the time.
- You can also get smartwatches that speak the time. Reminders can be set for taking medications.
- Get a big wall calendar, and at the end of the day, get your loved one to cross out the day. Notes can be made next to the date like, "Greg to visit." If your loved one still has a concept of reading, this will help them to anticipate visits from cherished people.
- As discussed before, signs can be put on doors and appliances to help them remember where everything is and what things are used for. If reading has become problematic, cut out pictures from a magazine to help establish what the rooms and items are.
- If your loved one is still able to get around, a walker with a seat attached (Like a Rollator) will be very useful. They can sit outside, following the sun. They can use the seat to transport things from place to place.
- If your loved one is still capable of speech, they may be able to use something like Alexa which has been programmed to switch on TVs and radios.

OVERCOMING COMMUNICATION CHALLENGES

It must be very frustrating to live in the world but to be totally confused by it. As dementia develops, your loved one loses the ability to think and speak, so communication does become difficult. Be observant so that you can catch anger, frustration, or agitation before it can fully develop. Make a note of what caused the upset and try to avoid that situation in the future. Of course, every day may bring another trigger, so when dealing with your loved one, you need to be alert in order to circumvent any potential threat to your planned day. Remember that every case of dementia is different. People are coming into it from different walks of life, different character traits, and different levels of education. There are also factors such as their personal history, gender, and race, so no two people will react in the same way. You may have been given some suggestions in your support group, but there is no guarantee that they will work with your loved one.

You are the reasoning adult in this situation, and it is necessary to keep your cool. Speak slowly, quietly, and clearly, no matter what is happening with your loved one. The force of their emotions may have scared them, so you need to talk them down off their personal ledge.

When dealing with your loved one, you need to take into account:

- The things that interested them before dementia became an issue. It is likely that they will still enjoy that, whether it be knitting, sewing, painting, playing a musical instrument, or singing. Build your daily activities on that.
- Their present-day abilities. You do not want to give them something that will frustrate them. If all that they can do is knit squares, that's fine; you can gradually build up a knee rug.

- Their memories can be used to build up a life history. This will be interesting for all family members. Encourage visitors to bring pictures or other memorabilia with them and let them build up a page together with your loved one, chatting about times together and whatever memories are held in their pictures or memorabilia. This will add meaning to their visits, making the time together enjoyable rather than awkward as verbal communication is getting increasingly difficult.

Encourage friends and family to make time for visits. A day in the life of a dementia patient can become very boring if outside stimuli are ignored.

COLLABORATING WITH HEALTHCARE PROFESSIONALS

At this stage of your loved one's life, it is essential that you, family, friends, and all manner of medical staff work together to afford your loved one the gentle care that they need. You will need to keep records of the visits to medical staff. You also need to be prepared to report on any changes in your loved one's condition.

The healthcare staff will probably be included:

- doctors
- nursing staff if your loved one is in a care facility
- physiotherapists
- dentists

In this way, your loved one's health care, dietary restrictions, and medications will be common knowledge to all medical staff as well as yourself, family, and concerned friends.

Your experience tells you that dementia symptoms will get worse. There may be good days that you can treasure, but unfortunately, your loved one is on a downward slope. As their communication skills decrease, you will have to step in to communicate with the medical team. You need to capture any medical issues so that you can voice your concerns with the team.

SEGUE

The communicating skills that you have developed with the help of this chapter are going to be challenged as your loved one's ability to respond correctly begins to create scenes. In the next chapter, you will learn how to handle these situations.

CHAPTER FOUR

MANAGING CHALLENGING BEHAVIORS

People with Alzheimer's can't change the way it makes them act any more than a cancer patient can keep the cancer cells from spreading.

— BRANDYN SHOEMAKER

People suffering from dementia often have to battle to understand their environment. Familiar places are forgotten, and people are strangers. The disease takes so much from them that it is inevitable that they will start to "act up." Your reaction to their bad behavior can either spur them on to be worse or help calm them down. If you get upset and start shouting, the behavior is not likely to improve. If you talk to them calmly and try to find out what has upset them, you will be in a better position to help them.

Always remember that their behavior may appear childish, but they are not children. They have been taught many years ago about acceptable behavior, but they are no longer able to express their frustrations in any other way. Words have been taken away from them so they only have actions to help them get what they want or need.

This chapter will help you understand why the behavior deteriorates and also what you can do to correct or manage the bad behavior.

UNDERSTANDING CHALLENGING BEHAVIORS IN LATE-STAGE DEMENTIA

Dementia attacks the personality in one of two ways:

- It could accentuate certain character traits, often choosing the questionable ones that the sufferer possesses. For example, if the dementia patient used to be short-tempered, they could become extremely irascible, flying off the handle the minute something doesn't go their way or...
- A character trait could be completely turned around.
  - A normal, quiet, even-tempered individual could become hot-tempered.
  - A man who has been faithful all his life may become a flirt.
  - A person who had extreme control over their home language could develop language that would "make a sailor blush," according to the idiom.

The behavior will probably get worse during stressful times like sundowning. Wanderlust also gets worse during sundowning. Your loved one could become agitated or restless. Distraction often works to get them to settle.

If they are experiencing pain but cannot find the right words, you may find that they resort to bad behavior in an attempt to be understood. This is a good time to use the cards to try to pin it down. Is it hunger? Is it pain?

Some examples of how behavioral problems could show themselves are:

- They will hide their precious belongings and then forget they have done so. The tantrums or accusations are rife. They will suspect everyone of stealing. Some of their hiding places are unique, and you will have to work hard to find the "stolen" goods.
- Their behavior may go the other way, and they can become apathetic and withdraw from socializing. Your attempts to get them out of their bad mood may lead to a fit of anger.
- Restlessness and pacing could lead to wandering. This is dangerous as they will get lost very quickly and could come to harm.
- Inappropriate behavior like making inappropriate sexual advances or disrobing in public can occur. There have been cases when a dementia patient has managed to disrobe and escape. They have been found disorientated and nude.
- They may start to hallucinate, which can be upsetting to you, the caregiver.
- They may become disoriented. This can be a very unnerving experience.

As a caregiver, you need to be strong during these stressful times, but remember that they probably have feelings that they are battling to deal with.

One of your best weapons during times like these will be distraction while you try to decipher what set them off. When you have established the trigger, you will have to ensure that that particular trigger doesn't happen again. Of course, there will be many other triggers, but calmness is your best weapon during these times.

Handling Behavior Issues

As communication is bad at this stage, you will have to explore other ways to find their triggers. Your loved one's body language may offer a clue. If not, try to establish what happened just before the incident.

Your loved one may be hungry, thirsty, hot, cold, or in pain. You can establish the trigger by using sign language or the cards. Maybe they just don't want to be in the space they are occupying. Take them outside or to a different room and see if this calms them down. Music will often help. Maybe try a sing-along of old songs like *You Are My Sunshine* or *Daisy, Daisy*.

Stress relievers like music, exercise, or indulging in a hobby may help get them out of the mood. Distraction techniques work well. They will not be able to see that their behavior is not appropriate, and telling them is not going to help either. You need to have tricks up your sleeve. A nice idea is a treasure box. This can be a cheap cardboard box or a classy wooden one. Fill it with treasures like buttons, beads, costume jewelry, cards, small booklets, crystals, etc. Let them unpack it. Exploring the items will be a distraction.

Person-Centered Approach to Behavior Management

Most of the techniques discussed before will be helpful while your loved one is having a bad behavior moment. Be accepting of where they are at that specific moment. Try to boil down what caused the incident, and then you may be able to deal with it. If they feel persecuted (like if they feel someone means to harm them), reassure them and make it seem as if you are dealing with the situation. It harms no one if you accept their fears as real. It harms them if you try to get them to see the reality of things. Their trust in you may be damaged.

In a dementia caring situation, your loved one is the most important being, and all aspects of dealing with the behavioral situation must be done in a person-centered approach. In order to do this, you need to know your loved one well. You need to know their triggers. When you are with them, they should be your prime concern. How their environment affects them must be taken into account. As you get used to dealing with these situations, the guesswork fades away, and you get control of the situation a lot quicker. Your loved one needs your empathy; you need to make them understand that you feel their pain.

Communication and Redirection Techniques

When your loved one has behavioral issues, be calm when dealing with them. Speak slowly and clearly, giving time for them to absorb what you are saying and to hopefully respond. Actively listen when (or if) they reply. Show that you are invested in their welfare. Use appropriate body language, maybe touching their hand or arm to gain their concentration. Make sure that your facial expression reflects your care.

Once you have their attention, you can redirect them to a more appropriate activity. Remember that their memory of recent events is shaky, so if they do not know what set them off, drop the subject. In the long run, it really does not matter what set them off, but if you can cast your mind back, you might get a clue when they cannot verbalize or remember the event.

Another thing that you need to remember is that your loved one's reality will not be your reality. It will be difficult for you to put yourself in their shoes as you don't know what they have perceived. It might be a real, legitimate issue, or it might be a perceived one—a hallucination or an irrational fear. You need to forget your perceptions and recognize that what happened to trigger the behavior problem was very real to them.

If you battle to understand what caused the present state of behavior, then check that the environment is not too hot, not too cold, not too noisy, or if there is too much going on.

Pharmacological and Alternative Interventions

At times, you may need to consider other solutions for your loved one. These can be medically prescribed or you could choose to try an alternative medicine.

Pharmacological Intervention

As we know, there are no drugs to cure dementia, but there are certain solutions that could help in behavioral situations. They will also enhance the quality of life.

- The most common type of drug is in the family of Cholinesterase inhibitors. The three makes of Cholinesterase Inhibitors are very similar, so your doctor might be guided by cost, sensitivity, and availability. If one make doesn't prove to be good then the doctor may try one of the others.
- Memantine is prescribed less frequently but may help your loved one. The biggest issue with this one is that people with kidney problems are advised to be cautious.

- Risperidone might be useful in treating your loved one's aggression, but there is a danger that your loved one may encounter unpleasant side effects.
- Laboratories are continually searching for the miracle drug for dementia sufferers. The discovery may be days or years away.

Alternative Medication

A lot of alternate solutions have not been studied for full efficacy. Most will be harmless and may assist, but some may need the approval of your doctor.

- **Aromatherapy** is a safe choice. There are many oils that are calming, like chamomile, rosemary, bergamot, lemon balm, and lavender. These could be used in a diffuser, but rubbing lavender on the temples could calm your loved one. Do not use undiluted unless the bottle says it is fine. You can use coconut oil or almond oil to dilute it. Chamomile makes a soothing tea. You could make a little bag to hold rosemary or lavender leaves that could be worn around the neck or wrist. Agitating the bag will produce a calming scent.
- **Music therapy** has been discussed and will certainly be a way to distract and calm your loved one.
- **Massage therapy** may be suitable as long as your loved one allows touching. Reiki could also be tried.
- **Pet therapy** could work with animal lovers. This has also been discussed previously.
- The use of **cannabis** is still in an uncertain position. Although many places in the world have legitimized its use, there are still many places where it is considered illegal.

Additional Techniques and Approaches

Boredom could lead to bad behavior, so all the activities suggested previously could be used to prevent boredom and other incidents.

Although boredom is not the only cause of behavioral issues, distraction works well with most. Just make sure that you switch the activities around, as you do not want to deal with boredom. To recap distraction techniques:

- The photograph album or scrapbook can be used to kindle memories of forgotten times. This could also be a time to bring out the treasure box.
- Drawing, painting (even painting by numbers), and playing with plasticine will bring out a creative side and stop the tantrums.
- Music, singing, and dancing will steer those behavior demons out the door.

P.J. and His Wife

P.J. was diagnosed with dementia after discovering that many familiar things and places were alien to him. Most of us know the feeling of going into a room and forgetting why we went there, but one morning, P.J. went into the kitchen and didn't know what the room was. He didn't know what happened in the room, what was stored in the room, or why the room was there at all. This concerned both him and his wife. On another occasion, he found himself staring at a funny "machine" in a wall, holding a (to him) random piece of plastic. He didn't know that the "machine" was an ATM and the plastic was his bank card. The people in the queue behind him were making random, not-so-nice comments, and he didn't understand why they were angry with him.

Soon after his diagnosis of vascular dementia, he and his wife started attending a sing-along for dementia sufferers. He had always loved singing, and his days started to be meaningful again. Music helped calm him when things got too stressful.

SEGUE

It is important to remember that bad behavior is not your loved one's choice. There is so much that has been taken from them, and their ability to express themselves leads to frustration. This frustration will normally be the precursor of a bad behavior episode. This chapter has hopefully given you more of an understanding of why they act up, as well as techniques to help you when this happens. Just know that your loved one may have more or fewer episodes than someone else, their triggers will be different, and their mode of bad behavior will also be different. But also understand that it is not something peculiar to your loved one.

The next chapter will deal with nutrition and hydration. You will be excused from thinking that no one can forget such basic functions, but the dementia brain has forgotten a lot of normal activities.

PREPARING CAREGIVERS FOR NEW CHALLENGES

One person caring about another represents life's greatest value.

— JIM ROHN

Caring for someone with dementia is filled with challenges from the very beginning. You might remember how you felt when your loved one first received their diagnosis, which may have been when their symptoms were still quite mild. Of course, your journey is unique, but it's very common for people to feel fear, sadness, confusion, and a sense of loss when they first hear the word "dementia." You may have sought information to understand more about what that diagnosis meant and what you'd need to do to take care of your loved one. But you're at a new stage of your journey, and what you're dealing with now is even more challenging than what you were dealing with then.

There's an increasing number of resources introducing dementia and caregiving to those who find themselves thrust into the role—and rightly so: As you may recall, it's thought that 75% of caregivers have a close personal connection to the person they're taking care of, and many of them have little to no experience. What's missing is the information about the changes that happen in the later stages of dementia and how caregivers can prepare themselves to handle them, both emotionally and practically. This book is designed to fill that gap, and it's something everyone in your position needs.

Your loved one either has late-stage dementia, or you know it's coming and you've decided to prepare yourself in advance; either way, you know just how much more is needed at this stage, and you know that other caregivers need this preparation too. This is your chance to make sure they have it. If you'd be willing to take just a few minutes to leave your feedback online, you'll help other people find this information more easily.

By leaving a review of this book on Amazon, you'll make it more visible to the people who are looking for information on late-stage dementia caregiving specifically, connecting them with the guidance they need much more quickly.

It's reviews that help books to reach their intended audience, and a few sentences from you will make a huge difference to other people as they seek advice specific to this stage of their caregiving journey.

Thank you so much for your support. No one is ever fully prepared for this role, but if we work together, we can make the road a little easier for the people who follow behind us.

Scan the QR code below

CHAPTER FIVE

NUTRITION AND HYDRATION IN LATE-STAGE DEMENTIA

Do what you can, with what you have, where you are.

— THEODORE ROOSEVELT

Both nutrition and hydration are important in maintaining good health at any stage of one's life. As your loved one enters the late stages of dementia, it becomes increasingly difficult for them to realize that they are, in fact, hungry or thirsty. This places the onus on you to ensure that they eat and drink at specific times.

Dehydration can play mind games and have other more serious implications. Your properly hydrated body normally has a blend of minerals, which allow for good performance. A dehydrated body will cause those minerals to become imbalanced, and this imbalance could lead to many health issues. As Mary was entering the late stages of dementia, she stopped taking in fluids. This went unnoticed until she became extremely disoriented, and all the other dementia symptoms went into overdrive. Fortunately, a doctor realized that the cure was simple. After downing a couple of glasses of water (protesting all the while), Mary was back to her old self again.

When you think of malnutrition, you will almost certainly bring to mind those horrific pictures of malnourished children in poor countries. You might be horrified to learn that your loved one is, in fact, suffering from malnutrition because they have "forgotten" to eat. It is strange that a person who is malnourished will lose interest in eating, but that is a symptom of being malnourished. A person who has stopped eating needs to be fed small amounts frequently until the condition is rectified. It will then be up to you to ensure that they eat three or four meals per day.

While nothing can be done to reverse dementia, it is comforting to know that you can reverse the effects of dehydration and malnutrition. By the end of the chapter, you will have more knowledge and techniques to help you and your loved one overcome the effects of both.

UNDERSTANDING THE CHALLENGES OF EATING AND DRINKING IN LATE-STAGE DEMENTIA

As dementia grabs hold of your loved one in these late stages, they will battle to coordinate their hand to bring food or drink to their mouth. They will need help eating and drinking. There are other reasons why your loved one may not want to eat:

- As their inability to deal with normal situations becomes worse there may be a difference in their routines. If they had always had lunch after a sing-along, and now suddenly there is no sing-along anymore, they could feel that lunchtime hasn't arrived yet. Remember, they will also be having difficulty interpreting body needs.

- Depression could take their appetite away. Any decrease in appetite should be examined for possible depression. If they were formally quite sociable and now they seem to sit for hours by themselves, they could be very lonely, which could lead to depression.
- A simple thing like dehydration could affect their appetite as well as cause other symptoms.
- The physical action of chewing and swallowing may be difficult. If they have dentures, get them checked to make sure that they fit properly. However, in dementia, your loved one may even forget how to chew and swallow. It may be time to consider other means of getting nutrition into their bodies. It is not uncommon at this stage to be fed via a tube. It is also possible that their throat has constricted, which could lead to choking while they try to swallow.
- As their lifestyle has become more sedentary, their body does not need as much to sustain it. Their appetite would decrease, but as long as they get enough nourishment to sustain life, it should be fine.
- Dementia may affect their taste buds and their sense of smell, so some of their favorite foods can no longer be tolerated. You will need to explore other foods, maybe even some that they positively disliked in the past.
- And finally, it could be that the idea of food is no longer appealing.

Identifying Signs of Malnutrition and Dehydration

The loss of appetite of your loved one can be worrying, but as long as their body is getting enough nutrition, a decrease in appetite is not problematic. Still, it is an indication that you need to ensure that they are not malnourished.

Some of the signs you could notice to indicate that your loved one is malnourished are:

- Walking and even standing may be too much for your loved one. If you have not personally supervised their intake, make searching inquiries to establish if your loved one has been eating.
- Weakness could develop into fatigue very quickly, where all they want to do is lie down.
- There will be weight loss as well. This may be difficult to pick up immediately as it takes a while for the loss to be seen just by looking. It might be an idea to keep a check on your loved one's weight about once a week.
- As the malnutrition grows, your loved one's immune system will start failing. It is important that you rectify the signs before this happens, as it will take a long time to build them up again, and they may be exposed to formidable germs in the interim.

Dehydration is becoming a real problem with many otherwise healthy people as well as those who are ailing. The fitter ones will get involved with a task to the exclusion of everything else and will forget to drink. Those with dementia will not forget to drink because that part of the brain has been damaged, and they can no longer tell if they need to drink or not.

Some signs to look for in your loved one if they are dehydrated:

- If you find them staring uncomprehendingly around and they are more disoriented than normal, sit them down with a glass of water. If they refuse the water, you can offer fruit juice, tea, or coffee; although these last three are not

as good as a refreshing glass of water, it is better than nothing.
- They may have a headache.
- Their lips may be dry, indicating that they have a dry mouth.
- Their eyes may have a sunken appearance.
- The urine will be a dark color, and they may show signs of constipation.

If your loved one is dehydrated or malnourished, the symptoms of dementia will be aggravated. There could be bigger behavior problems, or your loved one may not want to get out of bed because they are lacking in energy. They may not show any sign other than being listless. If there is a detriment in their symptoms, particularly if it is rapid, then before looking anywhere else, see if they are only, in fact, hungry or thirsty and may not be able to identify it.

STRATEGIES FOR PROMOTING NUTRITIONAL INTAKE

One of the first things you can consider is to make eating and drinking an enjoyable experience, remembering that a person with dementia requires a more specific environment than others:

- Create a calm environment. If members of the family are fighting at present, then request that they cooperate or take their meals alone.
- Everyone should be comfortable at the dinner table. If your loved one needs feeding, anyone uncomfortable with it should excuse themselves from the meal.
- Meal times should be sociable times, but with your loved one, noise should be kept to a minimum. Conversation is acceptable, but a TV blaring in the background is not. Cut down on all extraneous noise.

- Keep your loved one's portion small. It is overwhelming to them to see an overflowing plate. This, of course, means that they should be fed several small meals a day. Some ideas for snack-type meals are:
  - some avocado with a slice of bread
  - eggs done in your loved one's favorite way
  - peanut (or other) butter on a slice of bread
  - cottage cheese on a couple of biscuits
  - veggie sticks like carrots, cucumbers, or little tomatoes
  - fruit cut into small bite-size pieces (if serving things like apples, be aware that there might be a choking incident)
- Try to keep all meals finger-type food if your loved one is feeding themselves. Make sure that meat is cut into very small bite-size pieces.
- Have a glass of water on the table, as some foods might need the lubrication of water to help your loved one swallow.
- Let your loved one (as far as possible) dictate when they want to eat. It might be more convenient to have structured meals at set times, but if your loved one is having food issues, you need to meet them.

Meal Planning and Preparation

Your loved one may have dysphagia—a condition that makes it difficult to swallow. If this is the case, you will have to make sure that all meals are easy to swallow. A few tips will be included, but you might be happier to consult a dietician specializing in senior eating. In any event, all meals should be easy to swallow and digest.

Make sure that your loved one is chewing their food sufficiently. Around 20 or 30 bites per mouthful is considered a fair amount of time. If you make sure that all food on their plate is bite-size, chewing and swallowing will not be too much of an issue.

If your loved one has dysphagia:

- Make sure that they are drinking enough. It is suggested that all liquids be thickened. If the liquid (or food, for that matter) is too thin, there is always a chance that it will be aspirated, which could lead to lung issues.
- Smoothies are a good idea, particularly for breakfast.
- Thick soups or pureed vegetables are another way to sidestep dysphagia.
- Eat sitting up as straight as possible. If bedridden, then invest in a bed that can raise the head. A La-Z-Boy chair is also a good investment.

In preparing food, make sure that either before cooking or before serving, all items on the plate are either easy to pick up or easy to chew. Your loved one tires easily at this stage, so protracted meals are not on the cards.

Always have a good supply of snack-type foods to fill the gap between meals.

Assisting With Feeding and Swallowing

Some aspects have already been covered, like making meals with either finger food portions or soft, thickened meals, as well as having a supply of snacks between meals.

Your loved one will be able to feed themselves with the finger food idea but may require assistance for the soup. There are adaptive utensils that you can buy or you may opt to feed them yourself. A quick internet search will help you find the place to purchase them. Nowadays, there are so many specialty stores that deal with online orders that it should be easy to find a supplier. There are spoons, knives, and forks that are easy to hold if your loved one has tremors. Non-skid plates and something similar to a sippy cup are also available.

If you are feeding your loved one, watch that they swallow the food correctly. More care will have to be taken if they are feeding themselves. You cannot leave them alone to get on with the job, as they may choke while you are gone.

The correct consistency of the food may appear to you to be guesswork. Well, it is, and you may find yourself experimenting until you hit the right consistency.

Hydration Strategies and Techniques

Your loved one has lost all concept of time, so expecting them to remember to drink is a bit unrealistic. A good suggestion would be for you to program hydration times into their day. You could set a timer to remind you to get your loved one something to drink. They may balk at drinking plain water, but you can make it a bit more interesting by using fruit floating in the water or changing the color of the water by infusing it with some fruit juice. Soft drinks contain too much sugar, which may disrupt your loved one in many ways, like behavior, or it may even create a medical issue. When tempting your loved one to drink, it will help if you have different liquids for them to try, like water, flavored water (either shop-bought or homemade), juices, and soups.

Continuous dehydration could lead to urinary tract infections, kidney stones, constipation, and even falls. Hospitalization for the elderly is most often due to dehydration. Some symptoms have already been discussed, but there are many more:

- Dizziness is already a worry for senior citizens. This could cause imbalance and lead to falls, which could have serious repercussions for seniors.
- Cramps are common with dehydration. These could be very painful and of the Charley Horse variety.
- Heart rate and blood pressure could be affected.
- Skin is loose. When a section of skin is pinched up, it will take long to move back into place.
- And lastly, convulsions could occur.

So, how much liquid is enough? Daily Caring has a formula: 1/3 of a person's weight in pounds is a rough "guesstimate" of that number of ounces. So, if you weigh 120 pounds, you need to drink 40 ounces of water a day (DailyCaring Editorial Team, 2024b).

Remember that some vegetables and fruit have a high water content, so if your loved one enjoys melons, cucumbers, or leafy greens, you can make sure that these are served with their meals. Other fruits or vegetables with a high water content are:

- strawberries
- oranges
- pineapple
- peaches
- lettuce
- broccoli and
- lettuce.

Promoting Independence in Drinking

When encouraging your loved one to drink more, always keep in mind other conditions that your loved one may have. If they

- are diabetic then you should keep sugary drinks to a minimum, only giving them when a low glucose level is indicated.
- are hypertensive you need to make sure that there is not too much salt in the beverage choice.
- have high cholesterol then milky or creamy drinks are on the forbidden list.

It is important for your loved one to be able to drink independently of you for as long as possible, even if it means getting straws, cups with lids, or cups that have a weighted bottom so they cannot be tilted over.

Smoothies are very refreshing and nourishing. There are several meal-replacement shakes on the market that aid in hydration and are nutritious. Just read labels before buying, as they may include ingredients that could be detrimental to your loved one's health conditions.

Addressing Swallowing Difficulties and Ensuring Safety

If your loved one is gagging or choking while eating or drinking, it is possible that they have dysphagia. If you suspect this condition, it is important to get your loved one to the doctor. If food or drink is aspirated during the choking fit, it could lead to a severe lung infection, which your loved one does not need at this point in their disease. The medical advisor has a few tests that they can perform to finalize a diagnosis. During the test, your loved one will swallow items of different consistencies while being X-rayed.

When a positive diagnosis is found, the following will be suggested for the future (Hegg, 2024):

- If your loved one is having trouble swallowing their medications, you can crush the pill and mix it into a thickish food like applesauce or chocolate pudding.
- The use of a straw is not recommended as the liquid may travel too fast for your loved one to safely swallow it.
- Your loved one may have to forego treats like jelly or ice cream. The longer these stay in the mouth, the thinner the liquid becomes, and a person with dysphagia deals with thicker liquids better.
- While eating, encourage your loved one to sit up straight, as better posture makes the journey from mouth to stomach much easier.
- Spread the food intake over the day, giving several small meals rather than three large ones.
- If your loved one is tired, it will make swallowing harder.

All food textures should aim to be between very thin (like water) and very thick (like a stiff oats porridge). Solid foods will probably cause problems. As mentioned before, a smoothie could be your ideal solution.

Your loved one should be accompanied by a responsible person who can intervene if a choking episode occurs while they are eating.

COLLABORATING WITH HEALTHCARE PROFESSIONALS
AND CAREGIVERS

We have already discussed how to create an environment whereby you, your loved one, doctors, nurses, and so on will pull together to give the best possible care to your loved one.

When you have discovered problems with your loved one's hydration and nutrition, it is important that you discuss the issues with the medical team. It might be useful to keep an intake diary. You can detail exactly what food and liquid your loved one ingested, as well as make other notes that could prove useful down the line. You can start with the date then:

- On rising, make a note of what liquids they drank and how much.
- Breakfast:
  - What time did they eat?
  - Where did they eat (home, cafe, etc.)?
  - Make a note of what and how much food they ate.
  - Make a note of how much (and what) they had to drink.
  - Make a note of how they felt before and after eating.
  - Check for food sensitivities. These may only appear after a day or so, so you might need to go back to the diary if you pick up any tummy or skin irregularities.
- Morning tea—check the same sections as for breakfast.
- Lunch (as for breakfast)
- Afternoon snack (as for Breakfast)
- Dinner (the same again)
- And finally, before bed, drink and/or snack.

If you do this religiously every day, you will have a fountain of knowledge to share with your healthcare professionals.

Adjustments, additions, and subtractions can be done very easily when a complete record is kept.

SUPPORT FOR CAREGIVERS

If you are a family caregiver, you might be entering into this fairly blind. There are many courses in which you can enroll. Many of these courses are online and can be done in your own time. You can also get help from one of the many websites dealing with dementia.

If you wish to become a caregiver as a job, you will need some qualifications. If you already have a medical qualification, that should be sufficient, but if you do not have one, you will have to get certification following one of the many available courses.

It is a good idea to seek out people in a similar position. As mentioned previously, "a problem shared is a problem halved." This becomes very important if you are hovering on the edge of burnout—a condition that is very common for family caregivers. Check the symptoms below, and if you have a few of them, be warned that you need to start taking care of yourself to be an effective caregiver (*Caregiver Burnout* Clinic, 2023):

- becoming antisocial
- being physically, mentally, and/or emotionally exhausted
- finding it difficult to concentrate
- getting cross more quickly
- too listless to enjoy pastimes that you used to love
- suddenly feeling that the job is too much for you
- feeling anxious
- feeling frustrated

SEGUE

In order to maintain the best health in late-stage dementia, you need to ensure that your loved one is properly nourished and hydrated. Almost everything that goes into your loved one's system should have an element of nutrition. Make your mealtimes fun, something that you both can enjoy; just make sure that your loved one has finished the mouthful before saying something that could make them laugh or even just smile.

Financial concerns will be dealt with in the next chapter.

CHAPTER SIX

LEGAL AND FINANCIAL PLANNING FOR CAREGIVERS

We know the possibilities of growing old, but somehow or other, legal and financial aspects are often left too long. Fortunately, even late planning can help. If no one in your family feels up to the task of this type of planning and executing, there is help.

One family, when faced with the prospect of a life-threatening lung disease, found that they could get help with all financial, health, and legal concerns. These people are known as eldercare advocates and can be found via your insurance agents or even a Google search.

An eldercare advocate takes over and brings to fruition any plans you may have started making, as well as bringing many aspects, both financial and legal, that you have not yet considered.

This chapter will present many of the actions you, as a caregiver, will have to tackle.

LEGAL PLANNING FOR CAREGIVERS

Gather together all of the legal documents that your loved one has and keep them in a file together with any new documents that may be processed. This will help you keep track of them, and if you have employed a legal advisor, then you can hand the file over to them.

Some legal documents you will need to have are (*Making Decisions for a Person with Dementia*, 2023):

- Power of attorney (general) gives you (or another nominated person) the power to make decisions relating to many issues, including financial decisions.
- Power of attorney for healthcare gives you the power to
  - hire and fire medical staff,
  - decide on types of treatment,
  - find a suitable place for your loved one to see out the end of their days, and
  - make end-of-life decisions (including DNR—do not resuscitate).
- Durable power of attorney for finances and properties allows you to make decisions regarding any property of your loved one.
- Physician orders for life-sustaining treatment (POLST) will be drawn up in consultation with a doctor. The doctor's signature on the generated list will be placed in the patient's folder and must be available in the event that your loved one needs an ambulance or hospitalization. The agreements in the POLST must be followed regardless of any verbal suggestions you wish to give.
- A living will is drawn up by your loved one as it specifies what treatment they wish to receive at the end of life. As it

is drawn up with your loved one, it is essential that this is done before the disease takes too much from them.

- A standard will is also drawn up by your loved one. Most people will have a will, but it is good to make sure of this before the disease progresses too much.

- A living trust is important if your loved one has business interests and physical property that need to be managed. A trustee and a stand-in trustee must be named as the person they wish to take over their businesses and property.

- Guardianship will be given by a court if your loved one has not prepared sufficiently for the time that they can no longer make decisions so if you have the other steps in line, guardianship will not be needed. Guardianship will be needed if there is infighting among the people who stand to benefit from the death of your loved one. Unfortunately, this happens more than it needs to.

As most of us are not really up to scratch with legal issues, it will be best if you retain the help of a lawyer or eldercare advocate to get these documents ready. This is particularly necessary if there are many siblings involved, as well as if your loved one had a lot of property to leave. You want to make sure that everything goes to the person/s according to your loved one's wishes.

For American Readers

The following steps for obtaining guardianship are specific to American law and may be different in other countries, although the basic steps should be similar. The best advice is to discuss this with an attorney or the Clerk of the Superior Court's Office.

You will need to get a doctor's letter to take to the court, who will decide if you are a fit person to be the guardian. The court will appoint legal counsel for your loved one. That counselor will represent the best interest of your loved one, who will not be in a position to give any evidence.

If you think you need help getting your loved one to stop driving or to move into a care facility, you will need to get guardianship for them. If you have made sure that you have all the relative power of attorneys, your position as a carer (or guardian) will be easier to decide.

The first hurdle will be getting them to a doctor who can assess their situation and make recommendations. Your loved one may not want to cooperate with this. If they really dig their heels in, then you may have to ask the court to order them to see a doctor. All of this could result in an unpleasant relationship, so before embarking on this, you need to be sure that that is the road you want to take.

Getting that doctor's letter or recommendation will make things easier. Once the letter has been filed into the court's records, you will be examined to see if you are fit to be a guardian:

- They will examine your police record.
- If that is clear, they will examine your financial situation
- And finally, any conflict of interest must be resolved.

You are required to let your loved one know what route you are taking. This is not optional. Other interested parties, like family members, must also be informed of your intentions.

Once the court has appointed a lawyer for your loved one, a decision will be reached. The lawyer may require additional help. The lawyer is known as the attorney ad litem. If another person is required to assist, he is known as the guardian ad litem. Both of these will act in the best interest of your loved one. The attorney's job will be to advise and guide your loved one through the legal intricacies, and the guardian's job is to make sure that your loved one's interests are protected throughout.

Healthcare Directives and End-of-Life Planning

If you and your loved one have not had a discussion about how they would like to live out their last days, then it might almost be too late. If you have to make this decision by yourself, keep in mind all that you know of your loved one to ensure that their last days are as comfortable as possible.

By now, you have hopefully sorted out the living will and durable power of attorney, as these form a good basis for health care directives. Add to this (National Institute on Aging, 2022):

- A DNR (do not resuscitate) order. This will be put into force if there is nothing further that can be done for your loved one. This means that all forms of resuscitation must not be used. They cannot be given CPR or be Intubated. The doctor can make them comfortable but cannot do anything to prolong their life.
- A DNI (do not intubate) order means that your loved one cannot be put on a ventilator to help their breathing.
- A DNH (do not hospitalize) order means that your loved one will end their life in their own familiar surroundings.
- A POLST (physician order for life-sustaining treatment) order is a form that allows you to specify the type of treatment your loved one wants at the end of life.
- A MOLST (medical order for life-sustaining treatment) acts in a similar way to a POLST order.

- Organ, tissue, or brain donation can be mentioned. A brain donation could help doctors in their search for a cure for dementia.

Forms for many of the above are available. Some states or countries may not have forms for these conditions, but a form prepared by you and signed by your loved one in the presence of a witness may help. An eldercare advocate will prove to be helpful in locating and/or completing these issues.

However it is done, make sure that you have a copy on hand at all times and furnish all medical attendees with a copy.

FINANCIAL PLANNING FOR CAREGIVERS

Your loved one's finances must be handled by you or some other responsible person. If there is any doubt as to who should deal with the finances, your eldercare advocate will help with the decision. The following are things that need to be addressed:

- It will make it easier if all regular payments are made automatically.
- Any money coming in needs to be paid directly into your loved one's account.
- As checks are no longer as popular as they were previously, it might be an idea to swap to EFT for all transactions.

These three points will make it easier for whoever is managing the money. Don't forget to clear all of the above with your legal advisor. It may be necessary for your loved one to formalize things with legal documents that your loved one can sign in the presence of the attorney and a witness. This will give the nominated person a Financial Power of Attorney.

You, or whoever takes over managing the finances, should also ask your loved one how they want the business end to be handled. Some things to consider are how they normally manage their accounts:

- Do they pay in full or in installments?
- Do they give a regular amount to their charities?
- Are there any seasonal expenses that they normally cover, like birthday gifts?

If your loved one is not wealthy, the holder of the financial portfolio may need to examine other sources that could help with their income, like cashing in insurance policies that are no longer needed.

Long-Term Care Options and Funding

When your loved one is diagnosed with dementia, it is very likely that toward the end, you will have to consider alternatives to your caring for them (National Alzheimer's and Dementia Resource Center, n.d.-b):

- At the moment, you are giving unpaid care, but you may need to have some spare time as no one can be engaged in a job 24-7. Other unpaid help may be forthcoming from other family members or friends. However, you need to consider part-time paid carers as well. Chores could be:
  - cooking
  - cleaning
  - bathing

- ◦ entertaining
- ◦ transporting
- ◦ medicating
- ◦ shopping
- You will probably be spending most of your time with your loved one, so you are in an ideal situation to spot any anomalies quite rapidly. However, there will be other providers who need to be paid, such as doctors, pharmacists, laboratories, and other medical expenses like MRIs when necessary. Therapists may also be needed to help with movement or speech.
- If you take your loved one to a daycare center, there will probably be an expense attached to this, even if it is merely a donation. This is very important for your loved one as they will mix with others who are similarly affected, and they will be gainfully employed. They may play games and make knitted or crocheted items. They may also have singing and dancing or just movement exercises. There are some companies that farm out menial tasks like folding papers, stuffing newsletters into envelopes, and so on. This could be paid employment either to them or to the club. Either way, your loved one will benefit from the activity and the company.
- When it gets too much to keep your loved one at home, there are many well-run places that will take them in and provide them with assisted living. This is another cost that must be taken into consideration. The place will usually offer memory care.
- As things deteriorate, you may need to consider a 24-hour nursing home, hospice, or palliative care.

Cost of Care

Of course, there will be additional costs as no one other than you will be prepared to do it for love. The government will often have a program to help with the costs of care for dementia patients. You need to look into that.

Your loved one may belong to a medical insurance scheme that will have funds for their care.

They may have investments that give a small amount of payment every month, quarter, or year. If this is not considered financially viable, it might be an idea for the financial person to consider closing the investment and securing a bank account that will offer better terms.

If your loved one was a veteran, then they may be able to secure some benefits and possibly free or cheaper consultations and medications.

Of course, all this planning may have been better in the early stages, but you could still get help from many quarters.

Estate Planning and Asset Protection

There is no better time to encourage your loved one to consider planning for a future where they may have to move out of the family home. This is usually not taken well, and you may need to get the help of an eldercare advocate to help convince them that the move was necessary for their well-being.

Remember that apart from having their memory affected, your loved one's communication abilities will also be affected. Their ability to understand logic will also be affected, but despite all of this, you need to involve them in any decisions that are made. The only problem is that they may not remember agreeing to anything.

Your role as carer means that you will help your loved one make decisions and you will encourage them to stay informed about their finances and legal agreements.

SEEKING PROFESSIONAL ASSISTANCE AND RESOURCES

It will be almost impossible to deal with the topics in this section without the help of professionals. There is just too much to consider, and unless you have been involved in studying the ins and outs, you will quickly become bogged down. This is also where your eldercare advocate would be of great assistance to you. They will know which professionals are needed and will be able to suggest a few names.

- Attorneys (lawyers/counselors) will help you with the legalities of making a will, a living will. They can give advice about the various "do not" orders (e.g. DNR).
- Financial planners will help you get the necessary permissions if you are taking over the financial responsibilities.

Eldercare Advocate

If you feel you are sinking in the seas of finances and legal issues, you will need an eldercare advocate. If you find a few people in your searches, there are certain things you need to keep in mind before employing them (Hill, 2018):

- Set up a meeting where you can chat and assess if they will be a good fit for you and your loved one. This is like an interview and is best done face-to-face. Employing Zoom or Google Meet may help, but a person-to-person interview is much better. If you are lucky, they will be prepared to have a short interview at no cost.

- Before the interview, make a list of things that concern you. One thing may be how quickly they will be able to respond to your queries. Things that may affect this are:
  - How far away are they if you need a physical visit?
  - What is their experience?
  - How many similar clients do they have?
  - Do they have any referrals?
  - What do they charge?
- During the interview:
  - Ask how much experience they have in eldercare. Have they been in it for enough time to know the ropes?
  - Are you comfortable in their presence? If not, they are not a good fit for you.
  - Did they talk down to you? The way they address issues says a lot about them. If they explain things in an easy-to-understand manner, they are a keeper.
  - Take notes, as you may not remember the first interview after you have seen five others.
- After the interview:
  - You can review and summarize each person's responses
  - Do some research on them. Social media could be a good place to start.

A Strong Support System

A strong support system will

- give you the confidence to look after your loved one to the best of your ability

- and help you to cope when faced with a difficult loved one.
- steer you away from a possible breakdown.

Of course, your support system of family and friends is important, as has already been discussed, but a professional support system will keep you from drowning in legalese and spreadsheets.

Community Resources and Support

If you have enrolled your loved one in a daycare program or if your loved one is in a care facility, you may get help from the staff there, who could either give you advice or steer you in the right direction to get professional help. They may even know where you can get legal or financial aid at no or at least minimal cost.

It will be an idea to talk to other caregivers who can give recommendations and just be there if you need a shoulder. You will also be able to give and receive strength.

That professional help could well be for yourself, as caregiving can be stressful and unforgiving. If you don't get help when you need it, your loved one is going to suffer.

If you have given up work or even just have taken a sabbatical, you may be faced with a drain on your finances. You may be able to get some government compensation. Your Eldercare advocate would be able to help you if this is a possibility.

The many websites that are devoted to Alzheimer's disease or other dementias could be your first strategy. There is a list of likely websites in the reference section of the book.

- Your local clinic or hospital could have a list of practices.
- Your local library may have a list.

- There are also dedicated caregiver social media entries as well as websites.
- The American Association of Retired Persons (AARP) will have valuable information if you are based in America like:
  - insurance options (this includes medical, long-term care, car, and life policies)
  - savings on health care devices like glasses, hearing aids, and mobility solutions
  - financial and legal services
  - technology support
  - leisure time discounts
  - fitness discounts
  - help with securing the home and environs for your loved one

SEGUE

It is very easy for most of us to feel uncertain when dealing with the legal system. The same goes for some of us when faced with financials. This chapter has hopefully given us all someplace to go to for assistance with these matters.

In the next chapter, we will be detailing some more help options for you as we discuss support systems and resources from which you can benefit.

CHAPTER SEVEN

RESOURCES AND SUPPORT SYSTEMS FOR CAREGIVERS

Doctors diagnose, nurses heal and caregivers make sense of it all.

— BRETT H. LEWIS

M was a caregiver for her father. Before dementia took him, the family home was a happy place. Mom and Dad had lived with M, her husband, and her teenage daughter. There was always someone at home as they had staggered work hours. So when M's father was diagnosed with dementia, no one could see a problem. Dad would eventually give up work, but there would always be someone home with him.

After a heavy day at work, M picked up her shift of looking after her father. At first, this was fine, but as the disease progressed, M realized that she was the only one to deal with her dad during those sundowning moments. She began resenting her dad and the other family members, and this set up feelings of guilt. She couldn't understand these feelings as she had never before been a vengeful person, but now she seemed to snap at the slightest provocation and become a screaming banshee, taking it out on whoever was near.

She found it hard to forgive her dad for this disease, even though she knew that it wasn't his fault. This brought up more guilty feelings. Fortunately, she started taking steps to learn how to deal with the situation and her guilt. While today, she admits she is a work in progress, she has developed an understanding of the illness, and she knows that her father is also going through a hard time. She knows where the road is leading her and hopes that all the classes and forums she attends will help her deal with her dad more calmly. She is also slowly learning to deal with her feelings of guilt.

Until M has a total handle on her situation, it helps her to know that most caregivers have feelings of guilt, stress, and short fuses. She is learning that on the days she goes to bed and can look back on the day and feel satisfied that she has done the best she can. She knows she has succeeded—for that day. At the end of the week, she can see that she has had more satisfactory days than days when she lost it. Satisfaction with the day's work is a lasting feeling.

The skills that M learns in her research will help her bounce back and encourage her to be more positive about herself and the job that she is doing. These are strategies that she can use in all other aspects of her life.

Some of the techniques that M has learned are:

- She doesn't assume that the day will go well. She will deal with issues as and when they present.
- She takes time for herself. She spends an hour or so each day doing something that she loves. Sometimes, this hour is before her shift with her dad. That helps to set her up in a positive mind frame. Sometimes, this hour comes at the

end of the shift with her dad. She uses this hour as a barrier between her caregiver time and her time with her thousand or daughter so that she will not bring the day's frustrations with her.

She has become more decisive, and she deals with her tasks efficiently.

CAREGIVER SUPPORT ORGANIZATIONS AND PROGRAMS

Caregiving can be a lonely job, particularly if you are the sole caregiver in the family home. Fortunately, there are many caregiver support groups and organizations just waiting to help you, offer advice, or just be a shoulder to unburden yourself. These organizations know that caregiving can be stressful, but they also know that it can be rewarding in spite of its challenges. Just know that your being there for your loved one is the best gift you can give them. Also, know that you are not perfect and that you will make mistakes; after all, you are merely human!

When you started caregiving, you did not know half of what you know now, yet here you are, ready and willing to give your best. You have learned a lot, and yet there are still things that you need to discover.

Americans are fortunate because they live in the hotspot of new discoveries and new understanding, and many organizations are dedicated to helping you with your task.

- The AARP website offers (*Caregiving Resources & Links for Support*, 2024):
  - advice on caregiving
  - a legal checklist can be downloaded
  - online support available

- a built-in Eldercare locator
- Alzheimer's support
- memory café database
- Caregiver Action Network offers:
  - tips for caregivers
  - a video Resource Center
  - tips to manage caregiver stress
- The National Institute of Aging offers:
  - services for home caregivers
  - long distance caregiving
  - aging tips
  - tips for caregivers care
  - long-term caregiving tips
- CDC offers
  - support for caregivers
  - tips on caregiving
  - help in creating a caregiving plan
- The National Alliance of Caregiving offers:
  - help to discover if you can get reimbursed for caregiving your loved one
  - tips on looking after yourself
  - caregiver resources
- The Caregiver Space offers:
  - a place where you can get advice, share experiences, and get help
- Caring Across Generations offers:
  - a newsletter
  - courses
  - a platform to share your care story

When you are at home alone with your loved one, it is nice to know that, with a few touches of a button, you will be able to get the help you need. If you find venues close to home, it will benefit both you and your loved one to attend courses and mixers and just generally get to know people who are in a similar situation to yourself.

Brother and Sister: J and F

Growing up in South Africa, the pair was very close and did lots of things together. Both enjoyed music, and F was particularly fond of singing.

When they were adults, they relocated to the UK, and their lives diverged. Seeing one another became difficult, particularly when J moved to Afghanistan, but family occasions brought them together again. As the years passed, J began to notice that F was sometimes not really present during their phone calls.

Fortunately, J was able to travel frequently to London on business trips, and he made sure to visit F when he did so. He noticed that she was having difficulty in doing normal household chores. J spoke to her GP, and it was decided to send F for some tests. The tests revealed Alzheimer's disease. Now, at last, they knew what they were dealing with. It was recommended that they get help in the form of an admiral nurse, A.

This proved to have been the best decision for J as the nurse was able to make arrangements while he was out of the country. A helped J get the legal advice he needed. She also helped him take over F's affairs, which was easy using the internet and various apps.

Government Programs and Initiatives

The National Family Caregiver Support Program was created in November 2000 by the U.S. Department of Health and Human Services. This program offers:

- information on all the services that you could use.
- help in getting these services.
- respite care when needed.
- caregiver training and counseling when needed.

Most states have a local Area Agency on Aging (AAA) where you can get help. You can find your local AAA in the telephone book.

If your loved one receives Medicaid, then you can inquire if you are eligible for financial support during your caregiving years. However, be aware that each state may operate a different set of criteria.

Online Support Communities and Forums

As you have come to realize, you, as a caregiver, need support. If you can't meet physically to get support, there are many online platforms where you can meet with other caregivers for support and shared experiences. Virtual support is always available, no matter if you live in Botswana or Cleveland. Most websites have a staff member on call 24-7, so no matter what time you need to unburden yourself, there is someone available.

When you join an online support group, you know that others are experiencing the same sort of issues that you are facing. So when you unburden yourself, you know that others will understand. In your daily life, unless someone has gone through the same experience, no one else knows the depth of your issues.

A support group will often give you a coping strategy that you had never thought of before, and sharing your coping strategies may well touch someone in the group.

A support group may work on a Zoom or Google Meet call where you can see others in the group. It may consist only of sharing experiences in emails. Another method of sharing information will be in social media via Instagram, Facebook, or X. A WhatsApp group could also be formed where you can post a query or share an experience. Replies could come in thick and fast with suggestions or appreciation for your tip.

A support group could also offer courses that can be done online in your own time.

There is something about group therapy that fills a gap that doctors, nurses, and other health practitioners cannot fill. In joining a support group, you have the following benefits (Mayo Clinic Staff, 2021):

- You can feel safe that whatever is said, you will not be judged.
- It will help you to get a grip on runaway feelings.
- The tips you pick up will make for a more successful caregiver experience.
- Your understanding of your loved one's condition will improve, which in turn will improve the time you spend with your loved one.
- You could learn about new, recently developed treatment techniques.
- You will learn about the various resources available to you, like health, legal, financial, and social resources.

There are a few disadvantages (Mayo Clinic Staff, 2021):

- Group members must stick to the group rules, but there is always a possibility that someone will try to disrupt or take over.
- As you don't really know the other members, you may be slow to share confidence. You may be scared that what you say will be repeated and gossiped about.
- Whenever a group of people gather together, there is always a possibility of conflicting views.
- Always check any advice given by a reputable healthcare person.
- There is a possibility of unnecessary competition like, "My case is worse than yours." or "My loved one is an angel compared to yours." You will need to take it with a bunch of salt.

Support groups should come with no strings attached. There should not be a joining fee if it is not a business; however, if it is run by a trained professional, there may be a fee attached. While products, medications, and treatments can be shared, there should never be pressure to buy or try.

Remember that you need to feel comfortable in the group. If some of the ideas or people do not sit well with you, then try another group.

Resources for Online Support

Many support groups operate on a closed Facebook page. This means that they are trying to block people who really have no right to be there. You may be asked a few questions before being allowed to share or even read posts.

It is easy to find these groups, but you will have to join Facebook if you are not already a member. Facebook has a search facility. Once you are in the search mode, enter the full name of the Facebook group. For easy identification, I have accented the group name (*Caregiver Support & Resources*, n.d.).

- *Memory People* is a Facebook-based group created by an Alzheimer's patient. It is a place to share your experiences and gain insight from other caregivers.
- *Dementia Caregivers Support Group* is also a private Facebook group devoted to caregivers of dementia patients.
- *The Purple Sherpa Basecamp* Facebook group was created by a daughter who was the caregiver of an Alzheimer's patient.
- *Alzheimer's and Dementia Caregivers Support Chat Group* deals with caregivers in a brutally honest way and realizes that humor can be used to help stressed caregivers.
- *Dementia Caregivers Support Group* was created by a primary caregiver and currently has more than 43,000 members.
- *Caring For Spouse With Dementia* is a useful Facebook group if your loved one is your spouse.
- *Caregiver Support Community* is a Facebook group for family caregivers rather than paid caregivers.
- *Caring for Elderly Parents* may be the right Facebook group for you.
- *Working Daughter* Facebook page understands where you are coming from if you are trying to hold down a job and care for your loved one.
- *Caregivers Connect* Is a Facebook group for family members.

- *The Caregivers Space Community* is a Facebook group for caregivers of elderly loved ones and has more than 7,000 members.
- *Caring For the Caregiver Support Group* is a Facebook group open to all caregivers, whether voluntary or paid.
- *Caregivers Hub Support Group* is a good Facebook page if you are new to caregiving. It is open to voluntary or paid caregivers.

There are some websites that offer a forum. A quick Google search will get you to them (*Caregiver Support & Resources*, n.d.):

- AgingCare's Caregiver Forum is an active forum on the *Aging Care*'s website. You can read through the posted Q and As, but if you want to post a query or comment you will need to join the forum.
- Family Caregiver Alliance (FCA) is an online support group offering advice for your loved one's dementia.

PROFESSIONAL SUPPORT SERVICES

If you have decided to care for your loved one at home for as long as possible, it will help if you know where to get the help you need when you need it. Home health care agencies will give you the support you need, whether it be skilled nursing all the way to just companionship. Using these services will give you a break to go shopping or merely to indulge yourself for a couple of hours. Most of us, particularly if we are in a caring profession like nursing or teaching, spend too little time on ourselves, and when we do, we feel guilty. There is no need for that. You have worked hard and deserve the time to pamper yourself once in a while.

These services can help with

- medical care, like dressing wounds, giving injections, or changing drips.
- bathing your loved one if you are battling to lift and transport them to the bathroom and then back again to dress them for the day or night.
- food preparation if you are not too good in the kitchen or just need a break. Meals on Wheels is an organization that delivers precooked meals for a small cost. You just need to find out if you qualify.
- physical therapy in your home. This is useful if transporting your loved one is problematic.

These services will help relieve your stress build-up while at the same time bringing variety into your loved one's life.

Respite care is another option for you if you wish to avoid a break-down from stress and being too busy. Taking your loved one in for a few days will give you a break during which you can attend to things that you have let slide. It will allow you a breathing space for yourself and your family. My advice to you is to find a respite home early on in your caregiving experience. In this way, you will have done all your research long before you need it.

M's Experience With Respite

Merriam-Webster defines the word respite as "to grant a tempo-rary period of relief to..." (Merriam-Webster, n.d.), and that is exactly what a respite facility does.

M was exhausted at the end of the day because of caring for her mom and her school-going children. You see, M was a "sandwich carer," sandwiched between her own family and her mother, who suffered from dementia. Sometimes, it was difficult to fathom who to give attention to.

Her sleep cycle was disrupted, and she barely had enough time to sort out her own hygiene needs. So, when a respite center was mentioned in her care group, she decided to give it a try. She found a nice center close to her home, and they had a vacancy coming up, so she booked her mom in.

The break allowed her time to recharge, spend time with friends, and rediscover her passion for painting. When it was time for mom to come home, she was met with a revitalized M.

It would be silly to gloss over the fact that M did experience some guilt, which resurfaced periodically during her break, but she had done her homework before choosing the respite home. She was given the following advice when she started looking for a respite home:

- Ask about their licenses and qualifications.
- Ask if they have any references. You may also get this from their social media page.
- Ask your support group/s if they have recommendations. Also, ask if anyone has had dealings with the one close to your home.
- What services do they offer? Is this sufficient for your loved one?
- Find out what their staff-to-patient ratios are. A 1:4 ratio is a good ratio.
- In an interview, are you happy with their openness? If they are open and you feel comfortable with them, then you will probably be happy with them caring for your loved one.

- And lastly (and most importantly), what are their costs? Does health insurance cover the cost? And do they have payment options?

Caregiver Training and Education Programs

One cannot dive into a caregiving position with no knowledge. Your loved one might have suddenly needed your care, and you might have had to dive in. If this is the case, And it probably is, you will need to become knowledgeable pretty quickly. Fortunately, your first port of call should be a support group as you can get quick answers to your problems, but there will also be others who have encountered the same problems and have probably written or chatted about it. But that shouldn't be the sole source of help.

There are many training programs available. The more knowledge you gain, the better you will be at your job and the more helpful you will be to newcomers to your support group. The Alzheimer's Association website has on offer (Alzheimer's Association, 2024b):

- *Dementia Conversations* will help advise you on
  - when to stop your loved one from driving
  - how to deal with doctor's visits
  - legal issues
  - financial issues
- *Effective Communication Strategies* will help you to converse with your loved one even when things get tough and verbal communication isn't possible.
- *Managing Money* course will help those of you who are a bit financially inept! The course covers:
  - costs of caregiving
  - how to plan early enough
  - fraud

- ○ legal issues
- *Understanding and Responding to Dementia* will help you understand what causes the issues in dementia. It will give key points on how to figure out what a person actually needs. This may be different from what is verbalized by your loved one.
- *Living With Alzheimer's: For Caregivers—Early Stage* is a three-part program to help you deal with problems in the early stage.
- *Living With Alzheimer's: For Caregivers—Middle Stage* is also a three-part program that discusses how to provide your loved one with the care that they deserve.
- *Living With Alzheimer's: For Caregivers—Late Stage*. In this two-part program, you will receive tips on resources to help you in this stage. Professionals and experienced caregivers will help you through the problems you will face in this stage.

There are also programs specifically for loved ones with Alzheimer's.

It is estimated that approximately 10% of caregivers get training, which means that the majority of caregivers are untrained. Training assists with the following:

- Caregivers enter the caregiving arena prepared for the task.
- On-the-job stress is alleviated to a large extent.
- Health issues are fewer when a caregiver learns how to look after themselves.
- They can learn how to give injections, which will help with medical costs.
- Lifting techniques will be addressed.

MENTAL HEALTH SUPPORT FOR CAREGIVERS

If your loved one is a dementia patient, then your stress is generally much more than that of carers of patients with other health issues. You are also likely to suffer at least one of the following:

- depression
- anxiety
- health Issues
- stress
- compromised Immune systems
- cognitive decline
- insomnia or other sleep issues

With training, the impact of these health issues will be reduced. You will also be able to recognize a condition before it takes hold.

If you do find yourself beginning to feel the effects of caregiving, you must take it in hand before it gets out of control and your care of your loved one suffers or you get too ill to care for them.

Help could come from one of these sources:

- individual counseling
- support groups
- online therapy sites
- medication

Also, remember that there are respite homes. Taking your loved one there for a few days may just give you the breathing space you need.

ADDITIONAL RESOURCES AND STRATEGIES

If you have had to give up your job or take a leave of absence (which will often be unpaid), you may need some funds to subsidize you and your loved one.

Financial Assistance

There are a few options that you can explore.

- **Medicaid:** If your loved one is eligible for Medicaid, you may be able to get financial help to install safety features in the home or even to give you payment. You may have to jump through a few hoops, but if the end result is financial help, the hoops will be worthwhile. Some states may want you to become a Medicaid provider. As each state will have its own variations, it is recommended that you contact your state's Medicaid. The program that they offer will often be termed a "self-directed service."
- **Veteran services:** If your loved one is a veteran, you can apply for assistance. This could either be a pension for your loved one or a caregiver stipend. You can contact them via their VA Caregiver Support line at 1-855-260-3274.
- **Structured family caregiving:** This will be offered through Medicaid to pay you a caregiver's allowance. There are certain conditions that need to be met:
  - Your loved one must be eligible for Medicaid.
  - They must need care 24-7
  - They need assistance with personal tasks.
- **Adult foster care in your home:** Some states will provide you with extra income, but there are some conditions.
  - You may have to receive training.

- ○ There has to be a backup provider.
  - ○ You need to be open to periodic, unannounced visits.
  - ○ You cannot apply if your loved one is a spouse.
- Social Security may have a program that will suit you.

Legal Assistance

Legalities have been discussed earlier, but there are still a few things that need to be addressed. There are several places that can give you pro bono advice. Some will do it via a personal visit, and others may do it telephonically or via an application like Zoom. Some advice offered by the American Bar Association (ABA, 2019):

- Know when your loved one is no longer able to make decisions.
- If your loved one is in a facility and you can't be their eyes and ears 24-7, be aware of signs of abuse and know when to take action against the facility or the responsible caregiver.
- Be in possession of all the power of attorneys that you need to be able to make decisions for your loved one.
- Always be aware of your legal authority. You may have some authorities that were date-stamped and are no longer valid.
- Be aware of what benefits you can get (as above)
- Some employers could give you leave to care for your loved one. This means that your job will be available when your duties are finished. Be aware of what your company offers. It might be unpaid, full pay for a set amount of time, or partial pay.

- If your loved one wants to financially compensate for your care, be aware of conditions that apply to that. Each state could have its own conditions.

Resilience-Building Techniques and Self-Care Strategies

One of the first rules of caring is to care for yourself. If you get sick, then your loved one may be stranded. Women seem to be particularly at fault with this. It is probably the mothering instinct that survives! But man or woman, care for yourself first.

Generally, the following are areas where you need to take care. (Family Caregiver Alliance, 2023):

- Make sure you get enough sleep. If you are tired, you will become crabby, but you will also be more vulnerable to any germs doing the rounds.
- Eat healthily and do not skip meals. Make sure that you get variety in your diet and get vitamins into your body, even if you use a vitamin supplement. Taking care of your nutrition will also make you stronger and less liable to catch bugs that are doing the rounds.
- Keep up a regimen of exercise even if you feel too tired; you need to exercise. This can be as simple as taking a walk with your loved one or doing Chair Yoga with your loved one. They also need the exercise unless they are specifically bedridden.
- If you are ill—stay in bed or at least stay away from your loved one. Lots of rest is needed, and medication if necessary.
- Don't put off checkups with your doctor. If you and your loved one go to the same doctor, book in for a double appointment when you take them to the doctor.

A lot of us may feel that it is selfish to put ourselves first, but we cannot be effective caregivers if we are tired, run-down, or ill.

You need to guard against negative thoughts like "I am not doing a good job." or "I'm the only one who can take care of them." Your brain is a funny thing and it will frequently act on these thoughts as if they were facts. So you might actually convince your brain that you are doing a bad job or that no one else can care as you do. This results in you feeling inadequate or pressured to be the best.

To take care of yourself, you will need to do the following (Family Caregiver Alliance, 2023):

- Reduce stress. Get help if you need it. Don't refuse assistance when it is offered. Learn to pick up hints that you are stressed. Realize what is causing you stress and work to eliminate the stress by addressing the issue that is causing it. It may mean that you need to change what and how you are doing things. Remember, you can change yourself, but your loved ones cannot change the effects of the disease.
- Set goals for yourself. These can be daily goals or even goals for where you see yourself in three months or a year. Once the goal has been set—work toward it.
- Seek solutions to issues. As the disease progresses, you will meet new challenges. Read up on it or chat with others who may have dealt with that issue.
- Watch how you communicate with your loved one. If there is a problem, do not say things like, "You make me cross when you do that." Rather say, "I worry when you do that." Note that in the first, you are putting the blame on them, whereas in the second, you are shouldering the blame. You are, after all, the stronger one in this relationship.

- Accept help or look for help. Many friends and relatives have probably offered help. Don't try to be strong and say things like, "Thank you, but I can manage." No, you can't. You need the help, even if only for an hour or so, or getting a friend to shop for you. Use delivery services to get food into the home.
- Listen to your mind. Your emotions can easily get the better of you. Learn to recognize triggers and deal with them before they become a problem. You might even consider professional help if you cannot control these issues.
- Set Boundaries. These are self-imposed boundaries as well as boundaries that others are involved in.

In all your caregiving, be mindful and stay in the moment.

- Mindful means be aware (Merriam-Webster, n.d.). Be aware of your loved one's comfort, moods, and pain. Be aware of your surroundings that may be causing behavior issues. Is the TV too loud? Are there mirrors that scare them because they think it is a stranger?
- Staying in the moment means whatever is happening, you give your full attention to it.
  - If you are watching TV with your loved one, remember TV is not a babysitter. Chat with your loved one, point out things of interest, and discuss the show immediately.
  - If you are playing a game with your loved one, give all your concentration to the game and help your loved one achieve success.
  - If you take your loved one for a walk, concentrate on what is around you. Bring your loved one's attention to the birds, flowers, or butterflies.

- ◦ Talk to your loved one when dealing with intimate tasks like bathing.

Takeaways From Other Caregivers

You may hear of many of these things in your caregiver groups:

- Keep communication open with your close family, like your spouse or children.
- Never be shy to request help.
- Caring gave a sense of purpose when other aspects of life were disintegrating. One carer had just gone through both a divorce and empty nest syndrome. She found that caring for her parent gave her a sense of purpose.
- Accept care and kindness no matter where it comes from.
- Adapt to your circumstances as your circumstances cannot adapt.
- Learn to balance your life.
- Talk about your situation. Somehow, we all tend to shy away from talking about brain disorders. We are not shy to discuss a broken limb, so we should not be shy to talk about dementia and how it is affecting us. If we don't talk, no one knows how we are coping, and no one can give advice.

PRACTICAL RESOURCES FOR DAILY CAREGIVING

Earlier in the book, we discussed the changes that could be made in the home environment to help your loved one. There are other things that can also help. It is better to start getting the changes done as soon as dementia is diagnosed. In this way, things can be staggered, and your loved one can slowly get used to the change.

Things to Consider

Your loved one may need assistance remembering things that are happening or things that need attention.

- While they are still capable of reading and understanding the written word, you could install a bulletin board in a central venue like the kitchen. Whiteboards are available in many sizes. Appointment times could be recorded, as could a list of activities.
- Large wall clocks will help them observe the time and maybe the day as well.
- Dosette boxes (pillboxes with compartments for the days of week, morning, and evening doses. Some are available with lunchtime compartments as well). You could also get electronic pill dispensers with a time alarm.
- Timers in the kitchen will remind them of food cooking on the stove.
- Grip extensions on taps are helpful if your loved one has trouble turning a tap on or off.
- Grab bars, non-slip mats, and seats in the shower or bath will help with bathing.
- Incontinence pads or pants can be bought for your loved one if they have trouble getting to the toilet in time. There are several makes of pants that are washable. Although the initial cost is expensive, they will work out cheaper than disposable pads or pants. They are also better for our environment.
- If your loved one becomes almost bedridden, you can install
  - a hospital-type bed.
  - pulleys to help lift the patient from the bed to the wheelchair.

- ○ ramps for wheelchairs.
  - ○ recliner chairs with a built-in lift to help your loved one stand up.
- For eating, there are non-spill cups and cutlery with non-slip handles. Crockery should be a contrasting color to the food that you serve. Mashed potatoes on a white plate may not be seen by your loved one.
- Wider doorways will have to be planned if your loved one is in a wheelchair.
- Avoid clutter and loose cables on the floor.
- Invest in apps for their phone, tablet, or computer that will be amusing but also encourage them to think. There are many coloring apps, word puzzles, and games.

SEGUE

While your loved one is still at home, you need to be able to finance the changes to the house and garden. If your loved one has funds and you have financial power of attorney, you may be able to handle the changes. It is, however, advisable to maybe hold a family meeting to discuss how to pay for this.

The next chapter will help you through "Palliative Care and End-of-Life Considerations."

CHAPTER EIGHT

END-OF-LIFE CONSIDERATIONS AND PALLIATIVE CARE

One person caring for another represents life's greatest value.

— JIM ROHN

The start of dementia could quite easily be ignored. A person steps into a room and has no idea what they came for. A person with an aging brain will remember in a minute or so. A person with the start of dementia will have no idea why they are there, and the memory will not kick in at a later stage.

As the dementia progresses, the memory gets worse, and other behaviors start to appear.

L's Story

L's mother had early-onset Alzheimer's. She describes how her last goodbye was just the culmination goodbye that she had been saying for years. At each stage, her mother lost something of herself, but she kept her intrinsic character even though she lost almost everything else.

In the beginning, she had found creative ways to deal with her mom's loss of memory, so when the final memory crunch came (and it came rapidly). Her words for describing the rapidity of the decline are, "It was as if we were meandering along and then, without warning, we just fell off a cliff" (Laury, 2019).

After the initial battle to find words came the wandering, and her mom would get lost. Fortunately, there always seemed to be someone around who could return her to her home.

At this point, it became evident that L had to consider rehoming her mom.

L describes the disease as cruel and insidious as she watched her mom descend into fear and aggression. She would walk around the facility, trying all the doors in her effort to escape. But then the walking stopped, all coordination went, and eventually, she could not even feed herself. At times, there was recognition in her eyes, but she couldn't identify L as her daughter, even though it was obvious that she knew that L was someone special to her.

L's takeaway from her experience was that when there is love, love will prevail. Even at the end, her mom was aware that there was a special connection, a special love that they shared.

UNDERSTANDING END-OF-LIFE IN LATE-STAGE DEMENTIA

Doctors can predict how long people can live with diseases like cancer and heart failure, but it is not that easy to predict with dementia. However, in the late stages, there are signs that can help them predict how much longer the patient has.

As your loved one reaches the end of their journey, you may find that the dementia symptoms begin to worsen. You will probably notice the following in your loved one (Alzheimer's Society, 2019a):

- Their immunity weakens, making them more susceptible to infections.
- Your loved one will become more frail.
- Their balance could get worse, making falls more likely.
- They will lose their desire to move around and will sleep more.
- Eating and drinking become difficult, and they will need assistance. They may even have to be put on a drip if their medical directives allow it.
- Their verbal abilities will decrease, as will their ability to understand you when you talk to them.
- They may have cold extremities.
- Breathing becomes more labored and rasping.

Your loved one may only experience some of these symptoms. There is not much that you can do for them at this stage except be there for them. Hold their hand and speak slowly and gently, assuring them of your love. Talk about memories and the hobbies that they enjoyed. Talk about family even though they may not comprehend who the people are. Make eye contact with them.

Surround the room with things they like, such as smells, actual items, or even music. They may respond to a gentle massage. You could put a few drops of lavender or rosemary on a damp cloth and bathe their forehead and cheeks with it.

Be aware of subtle changes in their expressions or hand movements. If they are whimpering, it could also indicate pain. They may be trying to indicate that they are in pain. Try to isolate the painful area so that the doctor or nurse can take suitable action.

Be aware of their environment, as this may be the cause of their discomfort. Ask yourself the following questions (Alzheimer's Society, 2024b):

- Is the room too hot or too cold? Adjust the temperature of air conditioners or take off or add blankets.
- Are they hungry or thirsty? Help them to drink or eat, but be careful that they don't choke. Choking could force the liquid or food into the lungs, which could then turn into pneumonia—a leading cause of death in late-stage dementia patients.
- Are they anxious? If this is the case, try to soothe them while investigating the cause of their anxiety.

Doctors can try to make them more comfortable with medications. This stage could last a few days or may carry on for a few months.

Your loved one may experience delirium at the end of their life. Delirium indicates a rapid decrease in the state of mind of your loved one. Because the symptoms of delirium are so close to the symptoms of dementia, it is often difficult to judge if your loved one is experiencing delirium, but these pointers may be helpful (Alzheimer's Society, 2019a):

- Disorientation leads to a very confused state of mind. This can be very scary even when you are at the peak of your health. Just imagine suddenly realizing that you have no idea where you are or how to proceed. Now double that at least, just to get some idea of what your loved one is feeling. You will need to calm them down using touch, voice, or whatever other means you have.

- Distraction means they cannot concentrate on what you are saying or doing. This could lead to agitation. There are many causes for this.
- Delusions appear when they do not trust you and think you are out to do them harm. It is best in these cases to call in reserves and get a nurse, friend, or other family member to sit with them for a while. You will almost certainly find that when you come back, they will be pleased to see you, having worked out all their distrust of someone else.
- Hallucinations could lead to distraction and delusion. When they hallucinate, they truly believe that someone or something is there, and generally, they may feel that the "being" is there to do them harm. However, one patient was looking at a picture of a scene with no living being in the scene, and he saw a cat walk from one side of the picture to the other. He found this amusing. They may be scared by the hallucination or amused by it.
- They could suddenly become withdrawn and uncommunicative. Just sit patiently at their side until they come back to you. You could spend the time while waiting to reassure them of your love and that you are there for them.

Dementia takes years to develop, but delirium can start within a matter of hours. Doctors can use drugs to help them with that hurdle—but only if their medical records do not include statements not to medicate with certain medicines.

At this stage, you are playing a waiting game where the end is something you do not wish for yourself. You need the support of your circle of family and friends, most of whom are feeling the same as you are. You are experiencing anticipatory loss at the moment, which is delayed grief as you consider the world without your loved one. Your time together through this journey has made you closer and given you a new meaning to your life, and you may feel that you cannot return to your old life. Once grief has worked through you, you will find it necessary to pick up the threads of your old life together with support from family and friends.

In the end, you need to be able to look back on all the good things that happened and know that you did everything you could to keep your loved one comfortable, and you did.

L and D's Story

L's mom, D, was diagnosed with early-onset Alzheimer's when L was 25. She felt at the time of the diagnosis that together they could defeat this disease but soon learned that she wasn't in control of things; dementia was in control.

She sums up her experience by saying that with dementia, you are constantly grieving. She missed her mom even though she could see her; her mom was no longer fully in her body. But every now and then, her mom's sense of humor would come to the fore, and for a few moments, she had her mom back.

She missed not being able to get advice, and when she shared the details of her day, she wasn't sure that her mom could comprehend what she was saying. She often wondered if her mom was inside screaming to get out, as this is what she felt at times.

She feels that she learned a lot in her mom's final years. She learned patience, as well as learning that she needed to give up the fierce control that she had felt at the beginning of this disease.

When her mom passed away, she wondered what she was going to do with the extra time; she felt robbed and displaced. But overall, she was pleased to have been present for her mom, and she reveled in the memories of the love and joy she saw on her mom's face when she approached her.

Her published story helped many other carers who had gone through the gamut of emotions that L did. They talk of the guilt, the loneliness, and the memories.

EMOTIONAL AND PSYCHOLOGICAL CONSIDERATIONS

It is an emotional time when your loved one is reaching the end-of-life stage. It is also a time when things need to be sorted if you have not already done so. Do you know your loved one's wishes? Do they wish to die at home? Do they wish to be buried or cremated? What sort of "send-off" would they like? If they are religious, do they want a church service? Do they have a preference for how the final goodbyes will be said? Do they want singing? Do they have a favorite hymn or song that could be sung?

You must follow their requests as far as possible. It might not be possible to let them die at home as they might have been hospitalized for a serious complaint. If they are in the hospital, surround them with familiar things and play music that they like. (You may have to use a cell phone or computer/laptop with earplugs if they are in a ward.)

Everyone deals with grief in their own way. Some want family and friends around them and others prefer to be alone or with one special person. You need to be prepared for a range of emotions like the following (Alzheimer's Society, 2021b):

- anger at the one who left or at God
- disbelief; you cannot accept that they have gone
- numbness could occur as you have been so busy caring for your loved one that you do not have much more to give
- regret or guilt for not having done more
- sadness is normal
- you may also feel relief—relief that the suffering has gone. Relief that your dedication is over. This is a bad one as this relief could lead to guilty feelings.

Don't be afraid to get medication if you need it to help you cope.

Practicalities

You will need to find a funeral parlor. The staff are used to dealing with raw emotions and will give you as much help as they can. You will need to decide if you want the casket present for the funeral. If you do want this, who will be the pallbearers? Family or employees of the funeral parlor?

If you have a lot of people who are unable to make the funeral, enquire whether the venue can livestream the service.

The death will have to be registered, but the funeral home would probably be able to do that or at least give you advice. Your loved one's doctor has to sign the death certificate, so they may be able to help you with this as well.

The lawyer who holds your loved one's will must be informed, so make sure you know where the will is lodged.

You will have to attend to changes in benefits by informing the pension company or other financial source.

At the end of the day, you need to be sure that you have honored your loved one's wishes.

Ethical and Legal Considerations

There are several things to consider here like:

- **Advance care planning:** It is very unlikely that your loved one did not have this in place; few of us do. If you need to make decisions about the care of your loved one, make sure you do it sooner rather than later. If left too long, they may not be able to communicate what they want.
- **Withholding or withdrawing interventions:** This depends very much on what your loved one wants. If you have done the various DNs, you should be fine to follow their instructions in the DNs.
- **Quality of life assessments:** an assessment that works on a scale of 0 to 10. It deals with your loved one's physical, psychological, social, and occupational well-being and is frequently used to measure a patient's life with a chronic illness like dementia.

Earlier in the book, DNs were discussed, namely "do not resuscitate" and "do not incubate," but your loved one may have other things that they do not want happening to them. If these are in place early, you need never be afraid that you are doing things they don't want. It will make it easier for you to make end-of-life decisions with these wishes in place.

PRINCIPLES AND PRACTICES OF PALLIATIVE CARE

Palliative care enhances the quality of life in the late stages of dementia. It offers support to all concerned parties. For your loved one, palliative care gives physical care and minimizes emotional stress. It is person-centered care.

It will help healthcare workers if you have all the relevant information about your loved one at your fingertips. A suggestion is to formulate a "This Is Me" document. This can include things like (Marie Curie, 2019):

- family member's contact details
- their spiritual beliefs
- their current medications
- names of doctors and other healthcare workers
- their expectations for care
- as well as all the other things discussed in this chapter, like the will, DNs, and so on

Symptom Management and Comfort Care

Palliative care will take care of many aspects, such as:

- pain management
- breathing problems
- sleep problems
- providing comfort
- managing anxiety, distress, agitation, and delirium

Emotional and Psychosocial Support

Palliative care does not just give physical care; It also provides spiritual care, noting when a patient may need additional support from an outside source, a spiritual leader. This leader may not necessarily be attached to any religion as religion and spirituality, although often used as synonyms, are not the same. Spiritual needs are (Marie Curie, 2022):

- discussing the meaning and purpose of one's life
- expressing love for family and close friends
- feeling gratitude for the small and large blessings that life has given you

When a person is faced with the end of life, they may (Marie Curie, 2022)

- have an urgent desire to mend broken fences
- complete unfinished business
- have a hard time coming to terms with the fact that their life is over
- feel scared of the future unknown
- feel that they are losing control

Palliative care staff can help in these situations, and if they can't help, then they have the necessary contacts to call.

You could help your loved one to reminisce over the happy times in their life. If they can respond, ask them questions about their life. Allow them to become emotional when necessary.

Everything you do for your loved one at this stage makes your connection more meaningful as you keep their dignity intact.

END-OF-LIFE DECISION-MAKING AND BEREAVEMENT SUPPORT

If your loved one hasn't made plans for life choices in the form of an advanced directive or documents that spell out choices in the event of them not being able to make decisions themselves, you will need to get them to do one if they are still capable. If they are not able to do this, then the final decisions will have to be yours or a combined decision from the family.

Advance Care Planning and Decision-Making

The decisions that you reach for your loved one are called an advanced care directive and will include the following (Alzheimer's Association, 2020a):

- Religious beliefs. This could include spiritual or cultural ways to deal with death.
- Types of treatments they would allow or disallow. These could include references to:
  - using feeding tubes when necessary
  - using an IV drip when dehydrated
  - treatment of infections using antibiotics
  - helping breathing by using a respirator and intubation
  - being fed by tubes
  - having necessary life-prolonging surgery
  - relocating to palliative care institutes

If there are no advanced directives, you hopefully know your loved one's wishes well enough to make their passing peaceful. Here are some guidelines to help you build up a care plan for your loved one. This will be done by you (plus any other concerned family members) and the involved medical staff.

One thing you will need to keep in mind is that dementia is a disease of the brain, and since the brain controls your body, dementia has physical repercussions as well. It has been said that the goals of medical care are to "cure sometimes, relieve often, and comfort always" (USC School of Medicine, 2024). This statement gives you choices. You have to decide which is more important.

Curing the disease is not, at this stage, possible, so that leaves you with choosing between relieving the symptoms or keeping your loved one comfortable and giving a good quality of life.

As you know your loved one better than the medical staff, they should be guided by you when choosing a path of treatment for your loved one. When choosing a course of action, remember that your loved one is not just a patient; they are a person with likes, dislikes, and interests, so you need to include some things that make them happy.

Support for Families and Caregivers

Families of dementia patients are often described as having *ambiguous loss,* a term used to describe the loss of a person while the person is physically still alive. As the disease continues and your loved one progresses through the stages of dementia, you may find the ambiguous loss turning into *anticipatory grief.* This is grief for a person who has lost their intrinsic being. You can see the shell of the loved one, but the person inside the shell will never come back to you.

Both of these conditions stop when your loved one dies, and the grief becomes the grief that we all know and dread. Grief is intense. For a while, a caregiver will feel the loss of their loved one in many different ways. The most obvious way is that the person is not there and will never be there, but the caregiver will also feel a loss of purpose and will suddenly be faced with far too many empty hours, hours that they had spent caring for their loved one. It is also common for a caregiver to feel insecure, not knowing where to go and how to get through the next days, weeks, and months.

No one grieves for the same amount of time. Grief is intensely personal, and no one should try to put a time limit on it. The way you handle grief is also personal. Some people are angry. Angry at your departed loved one, angry at your maker or the universe, angry that you are still here. If you are worried about how you are handling grief, there are Facebook groups and websites, and of course, you could get personal care by either joining a physical support group or having a few sessions with a professional. Just remember that your grief is personal and will probably be different from the way others are handling it, so there is nothing wrong with the way you are grieving.

Symptoms of Grief

I am giving you these symptoms so that you know you are not abnormal. You may experience one or many of the following (Family Caregiver Alliance, 2013):

- fatigue
- changes in appetite
- problems with sleeping
- loneliness and isolation from others
- feeling overwhelmed
- feelings of guilt
- depression
- helplessness
- unstable emotions
- not understanding why there has to be death
- reconsidering your faith

It is normal for people to go through stages of grief. First, there is denial, which is followed by anger and then bargaining with your deity. Depression follows, and then you get acceptance. Through all these stages, try to put yourself first and take care of yourself.

Coping Strategies

Don't try to stifle your grief; let it work its way through you. Try to talk to friends and family about it and express your feelings, whether you are feeling angry, sad, or hopeless. It might help you to write down what you are feeling. Try to keep yourself occupied, and return to work as soon as you can. Go for walks or attend an exercise class.

Just know that someday, you will find the memories that will help you heal.

SHARE YOUR EXPERIENCE

Caregiving can be a very lonely experience, and hearing from other people on the same journey can make a huge difference. Take a moment now to share your story with others, and let them know where they can find the guidance they're searching for.

Simply by sharing your honest opinion of this book and a little about your own experience with dementia, you'll show new readers exactly where they can find this information—and you'll remind them that they're not alone in the process.

WANT TO HELP OTHERS?

Thank you so much for your support. The more we share our stories, the more we can help others who are facing the same challenges.

Scan the QR code below

CONCLUSION

In the end, you tried and you cared and sometimes that is enough.

— ANTHEA YANG

This book has explored all aspects of late-stage dementia. It has given you, as a caregiver, emotional, psychological, and hopefully, helpful advice. It has dealt with the realities of dementia.

We have looked at case studies, and you may have found consolation in reading stories that you can relate to. Things that have been tried by other caregivers might have helped you in your daily dealings with your loved one.

You have worked long and hard to help your loved one. At times, you may have felt that it was too hard, but you persevered, and your loved one appreciated your dedication even when they couldn't verbalize it. Even when they became angry or agitated, you continued.

If this book has helped you, let it help others who are on the same journey by leaving a comment.

REFERENCES

AARP, October 28, U., & 2019. (2019, October 28). *National agencies, groups and organizations for caregivers.* AARP. https://www.aarp.org/caregiving/local/info-2019/national-resources-for-caregivers.html

ABA. (2019). *American Bar Association.* Americanbar.org. https://www.american bar.org

admin. (2023, May 13). *What are the 3 forms of palliative care.* Oasis Hospice & Palliative Care. https://oasishospice.us/2023/05/13/what-are-the-3-forms-of-palliative-care/

Allen, K. (2016, April 20). *Three experienced Alzheimer's and Dementia caregivers share their stories and lessons.* BrightFocus Foundation. https://www.brightfocus.org/alzheimers/article/three-experienced-alzheimers-and-dementia-caregivers-share-their-stories-and

Allen, K. (2017, July 7). *Caregiver training: What you need to know.* BrightFocus Foundation. https://www.brightfocus.org/alzheimers/article/caregiver-train ing-what-you-need-know

Allen, K. (2021, December 1). *On the Alzheimer's caregiver journey: Tips for managing guilt.* BrightFocus Foundation. https://www.brightfocus.org/alzheimers/arti cle/alzheimers-caregiver-journey-tips-managing-guilt

ALZ Magazine. (2020). *Losing Gene Wilder.* Alzheimer's Disease and Dementia. https://www.alz.org/news/2020/losing-gene-wilder

#StillHere – Five personal stories. (2012). Alzheimer Society of Manitoba. https://alzheimer.mb.ca/still-here-five-personal-stories/

Alzheimer's Research Association. (2020, November 19). *Former Ballerina With Alzheimer's Performs "Swan Lake" Dance: Super Emotional* [Video]. YouTube. https://www.youtube.com/watch?v=IT_tW3EVDK8&t=4s

Alzheimer's Association. (n.d.). *A romance that started at age 14.* Alzheimer's Disease and Dementia. https://www.alz.org/media/wi/documents/Spiegelhoff-profile.pdf

Alzheimer's Association. (2019). *Late-stage caregiving.* Alzheimer's Disease and Dementia. https://www.alz.org/help-support/caregiving/stages-behaviors/late-stage

Alzheimer's Association. (2020a). *End-of-life planning.* Alzheimer's Disease and Dementia. https://www.alz.org/help-support/i-have-alz/plan-for-your-future/end_of_life_planning

Alzheimer's Association. (2020b). *Personal stories of caregivers, families and professionals.* Alzheimer's Disease and Dementia. https://www.alz.org/wi/helping-you/personal-stories

Alzheimer's Association. (2024a). *2024 Alzheimer's disease facts and figures.* Alzheimer's Association. https://www.alz.org/media/Documents/alzheimers-facts-and-figures.pdf

Alzheimer's Association. (2024b). *Educational programs and dementia care resources.* Alzheimer's Disease and Dementia. https://www.alz.org/help-support/resources/care-education-resources

Alzheimer's Association. (2024c). *Home safety.* Alzheimer's Disease and Dementia. https://www.alz.org/help-support/caregiving/safety/home-safety

Alzheimer's Association. (2024d). *What equipment can improve the home of a person with dementia?* Alzheimer's Society. https://www.alzheimers.org.uk/get-support/staying-independent/what-equipment-improve-adapt-home-person-dementia

Alzheimer's Caregivers. (2023, October 17). *Ask the experts: Can a robotic dog be a companion for people living with Alzheimer's disease?* Alzheimer's Caregivers Network. https://alzheimerscaregivers.org/2023/10/17/ask-the-experts-can-a-robotic-dog-be-a-companion-for-people-living-with-alzheimers-disease/

Alzheimer's Society. (n.d.). *Communicating and dementia – useful organisations.* Alzheimer's Society. https://www.alzheimers.org.uk/about-dementia/symptoms-and-diagnosis/symptoms/communicating-other-resources

Alzheimer's Society. (2018). *"With Alzheimer's, you are constantly in a state of grieving": Loretta's dementia story.* Alzheimer's Society. https://www.alzheimers.org.uk/blog/loretta-dementia-carer-grief

Alzheimer's Society. (2019a). *Recognising when someone is reaching the end of their life.* Alzheimer's Society. https://www.alzheimers.org.uk/get-support/help-dementia-care/recognising-when-someone-reaching-end-their-life

Alzheimer's Society. (2019b). *Reducing and managing behaviour that challenges.* Alzheimer's Society. https://www.alzheimers.org.uk/about-dementia/symptoms-and-diagnosis/symptoms/managing-behaviour-changes

Alzheimer's Society. (2020). *The progression of Alzheimer's disease and other dementias.* https://www.alzheimers.org.uk/sites/default/files/pdf/factsheet_the_progression_of_alzheimers_disease_and_other_dementias.pdf

Alzheimer's Society. (2021a). *Communicating and dementia.* Alzheimer's Society. https://www.alzheimers.org.uk/about-dementia/symptoms-and-diagnosis/symptoms/communicating-and-dementia

Alzheimer's Society. (2021b, September 6). *Coping with the death of a person with dementia.* Alzheimer's Society. https://www.alzheimers.org.uk/get-support/help-dementia-care/coping-death-person-dementia#content-start

Alzheimer's Society. (2023). *Making decisions for a person with dementia who lacks mental capacity.* Alzheimer's Society. https://www.alzheimers.org.uk/get-support/legal-financial/making-decisions-mental-capacity-dementia

Alzheimer's Society. (2024a). *Alternative treatments for dementia.* Alzheimer Society of Canada. https://alzheimer.ca/en/about-dementia/how-can-i-treat-dementia/alternative-treatments-dementia

Alzheimer's Society. (2024b). *End of life care: communication and physical needs.* Alzheimer's Society. https://www.alzheimers.org.uk/get-support/help-dementia-care/end-life-care-communication-physical-needs#content-start

Alzheimer's Society. (2024c). *Person-centred care.* Alzheimer's Society. https://www.alzheimers.org.uk/about-dementia/treatments/person-centred-care

Anderson, J. (n.d.). *Jamie Anderson quotes.* Goodreads. https://www.goodreads.com/quotes/9657488-grief-i-ve-learned-is-really-just-love-it-s-all-the

Arch National Respite Network. (2022, January 4). *How do I get paid to be a family caregiver?* ARCH National Respite Network & Resource Center. https://archrespite.org/caregiver-resources/how-do-i-get-paid-to-be-a-family-caregiver/

BBC. (2024). *BBC Two - Inside the care crisis with Ed Balls.* BBC. https://www.bbc.co.uk/programmes/m0011hfd

Better Health Channel. (2012). *Dementia - behaviour changes.* Better Health. https://www.betterhealth.vic.gov.au/health/conditionsandtreatments/dementia-behaviour-changes

Better Health Channel. (2014). *Dementia - communication.* Better Health Channel. https://www.betterhealth.vic.gov.au/health/ConditionsAndTreatments/dementia-communication

BrainandLife. (2023, July 27). *How caregivers deal with anticipatory grief.* BrainandLife. https://www.brainandlife.org/articles/how-caregivers-deal-with-anticipatory-grief

BrightFocus Foundation. (2021a, October 4). *Being an Alzheimer's disease caregiver*.BrightFocus Foundation. https://www.brightfocus.org/alzheimers/resources/being-caregiver

BrightFocus Foundation. (2021b, October 5). *Alzheimer's disease: Managing caregiver stress.* BrightFocus Foundation. https://www.brightfocus.org/alzheimers/resources/managing-caregiver-stress

BrightFocus Foundation. (2021c, October 5). *Supporting Alzheimer's disease caregivers.* BrightFocus Foundation. https://www.brightfocus.org/alzheimers/resources/supporting-caregivers

BrightFocus Foundation. (2023). *Caregiving for Alzheimer's patients.* BrightFocus Foundation. https://www.brightfocus.org/alzheimers/resources/caregiving

BrightFocus Foundation. (2024, July 1). *Managing stress: Care for the caregiver.*

BrightFocus Foundation. https://www.brightfocus.org/alzheimers/publication/managing-stress-caring-caregiver

Brodaty, H., & Donkin, M. (2019). Family caregivers of people with dementia. *Dialogues in Clinical Neuroscience, 11*(2), 217–228. National Library of Medicine. https://doi.org/10.31887/DCNS.2009.11.2/hbrodaty

CareFound Home Care. (n.d.). *Dementia Care at Home*. CareFound. https://www.carefound.co.uk/specialist-care/dementia-care/

Caregivers, A. (2023, August 8). *4 things to know about music & dementia*. Alzheimer's Caregivers Network. https://alzheimerscaregivers.org/2023/08/08/music-and-dementia/

Caregiving resources & links for support. (2024). CaringInfo. https://www.caringinfo.org/planning/caregiving/caregiving-resources/

Caregiver support & resources. (n.d.). A Place for Mom. https://www.aplaceformom.com/caregiver-resources

Carpenter, C. (2024, June 28). *The family caregiver toolbox*. Caregiver Action Network. https://www.caregiveraction.org/toolbox/?_disease=alzheimers

Chow, C. (2024a). *6 ways to get seniors with no appetite to eat*. DailyCaring. https://dailycaring.com/6-ways-to-get-seniors-with-no-appetite-to-eat/

Chow, C. (2024b). *Why do seniors lose their appetites? 10 possible reasons*. DailyCaring. https://dailycaring.com/why-do-seniors-lose-their-appetites/

Caregiver burnout. (2023). Cleveland Clinic. https://my.clevelandclinic.org/health/diseases/9225-caregiver-burnout

Caregiving & grief. (2024). Hospice Foundation of America. https://hospicefoundation.org/Grief-(1)/Caregiving

Daily Caring. (2018). *Get help with long term care planning: Making financial, medical, and legal decisions*. https://dailycaring.com/arag-get-help-with-long-term-care-planning-making-financial-medical-and-legal-decisions/

DailyCaring Editorial Team. (2024a). *11 adaptive utensils and eating aids for hand tremors, dementia, Parkinson's, stroke*. DailyCaring. https://dailycaring.com/hand-tremors-adaptive-utensils-eating-aids/

DailyCaring Editorial Team. (2024b). *Dehydration in seniors: An often-overlooked health risk*. DailyCaring. https://dailycaring.com/dehydration-in-elderly-is-dangerous/

Dehydration symptoms and treatments. (2023). NHS Inform. https://www.nhsinform.scot/illnesses-and-conditions/nutritional/dehydration/

Dementia: 7 stages. (2024). Compassion & Choices. https://compassionandchoices.org/resource/dementia-7-stages/

Dementia UK. (2021). *Will's story*. Dementia UK. https://www.dementiauk.org/information-and-support/stories/wills-story-people-deal-with-trauma-in-different-ways-and-there-is-no-roadmap/

Dementia UK. (2024a). *Personal stories*. Dementia UK. https://www.dementiauk. org/information-and-support/stories/

Dementia UK. (2024b, April 19). *Jolyon's story*. Dementia UK. https://www.dementi auk.org/information-and-support/stories/jolyons-story-admiral-nurse-made-me-take-care-mental-health/

Department of Health. Victoria, A. (2024, July 17). *Implementation case studies*. Www.health.vic.gov.au.   https://www.health.vic.gov.au/older-people-in-hospi tal/supporting-information-for-older-people-in-hospital/implementation-case-studies

Desai, N. (2023, October 12). *18 signs your aging parent needs help*. Www.aplaceformom.com.   https://www.aplaceformom.com/caregiver-resources/articles/parents-need-help

Desai, N. (2024, May 22). *What to do when elderly parents refuse help*. A Place for Mom.   https://www.aplaceformom.com/caregiver-resources/articles/parents-wont-listen

Do's and don'ts of communication and dementia. (2018, July 19). Alzheimer's San Diego. https://www.alzsd.org/dos-and-donts-of-compassionate-communication-dementia/

Eason, H. (2024, January 2). *What is caregiver burnout?* A Place for Mom. https:// www.aplaceformom.com/caregiver-resources/articles/caregiver-burnout

Elizabeth. (2019, March 30). *Sharing caregiving stories and self-care strategies helps everyone*. Happy Healthy Caregiver. https://happyhealthycaregiver.com/shar ing-caregiving-stories/

Ellis, M. E. (2016, November 21). *What are the stages of Alzheimer's disease?* Healthline.   https://www.healthline.com/health/stages-progression-alzheimers#stage-5

Family Caregiver Alliance. (2013). *Grief and loss*. Family Caregiver Alliance. https:// www.caregiver.org/resource/grief-and-loss/

Family Caregiver Alliance. (2023). *Taking care of you: Self-care for family caregivers*. Family Caregiver Alliance. https://www.caregiver.org/resource/taking-care-you-self-care-family-caregivers/

Fazio, S., Pace, D., Flinner, J., & Kallmyer, B. (2018). The Fundamentals of person-centered Care for Individuals with Dementia. *The Gerontologist, 58*(1), 10–19. https://doi.org/10.1093/geront/gnx122

Gates, M. (2024, May 27). *Adjusting to living with elderly parents: Expert tips*. A Place for Mom. https://www.aplaceformom.com/caregiver-resources/articles/living-with-your-aging-parent-doesnt-work

Ghebrai, M. (2021, March 16). *23 best caregiver support groups online and in-person*. A Place for Mom. https://www.aplaceformom.com/caregiver-resources/articles/caregiver-support-groups

Groen-van de Ven, L., Smits, C., de Graaff, F., Span, M., Eefsting, J., Jukema, J., & Vernooij-Dassen, M. (2017). Involvement of people with dementia in making decisions about their lives: a qualitative study that appraises shared decision-making concerning daycare. *BMJ Open, 7*(11), e018337. https://doi.org/10.1136/bmjopen-2017-018337

Hallstrom, L. (2022, October 18). *The 7 stages of dementia & symptoms.* A Place for Mom. https://www.aplaceformom.com/caregiver-resources/articles/dementia-stages

Harrison, E. (2022, May 31). *Tracking diet behavior: How to keep a food diary for a loved one with dementia.* Seasons. https://www.seasons.com/tracking-diet-behavior-how-to-keep-a-food-diary-for-a-loved-one-with-dementia/2606198/

Hawk, T. (2018). *Tony Hawk shares his personal Alzheimer's story.* Alzheimer's Disease and Dementia. https://www.alz.org/blog/alz/october-2018-(1)/tony-hawk-shares-his-personal-alzheimer-s-story

The Health Foundation. (2016). *Person-centred care made simple.* https://www.health.org.uk/sites/default/files/PersonCentredCareMadeSimple.pdf

Health, S. (2021, February 23). *Sensory stimulation for older adults with dementia.* SALMON Health and Retirement. https://salmonhealth.com/sensory-stimulation-for-older-adults-with-dementia/

Heerema, E. (2018, January 10). *Pros and cons of doll therapy in dementia.* Verywell Health. https://www.verywellhealth.com/therapeutic-doll-therapy-in-dementia-4155803

Heerema, E. (2021, November 9). *The complete guide to challenging behaviors in dementia.* Verywell Health. https://www.verywellhealth.com/the-complete-guide-to-challenging-behaviors-in-dementia-97607

Hegg, J. (2024). *7 tips for seniors and caregivers managing dysphagia.* DailyCaring. https://dailycaring.com/7-helpful-tips-for-seniors-and-caregivers-managing-dysphagia/

Hill, A. (2018, September 21). *If you are a caregiver or even if you have an elderly loved one, you might need the services of an elder law attorney. These lawyers specialize in issues that affect seniors, such as elder fraud, estate planning, and more.* LinkedIn. https://www.linkedin.com/pulse/5-tips-finding-right-elder-law-attorney-april-hill

Hipp, D. (2024, March 14). *How to redirect a loved one with dementia.* A Place for Mom. https://www.aplaceformom.com/caregiver-resources/articles/redirect-a-loved-one-with-dementia

Hobson, G. (2023, December 20). *Managing dementia behaviors: Do's and don'ts from experts.* A Place for Mom. https://www.aplaceformom.com/caregiver-resources/articles/dementia-behaviors

Hood, J. (2020). *The benefits and importance of a support system.* Highland Springs.

https://highlandspringsclinic.org/the-benefits-and-importance-of-a-support-system/

How to deal with challenging behaviour in adults - Social care and support guide. (2023, April 11). NHS UK. https://www.nhs.uk/conditions/social-care-and-support-guide/practical-tips-if-you-care-for-someone/how-to-deal-with-challenging-behaviour-in-adults/

Inspiring stories. (2022). Dementia Researcher. https://www.dementiaresearcher.nihr.ac.uk/category/insipring-stories/

Late stage dementia. (2024). Dementia UK. https://www.dementiauk.org/information-and-support/about-dementia/stages-of-dementia/late-stage-dementia/

Laury. (2019). *Laury's story: "Mum became utterly lost in the fog of her own mind."* Alzheimer's Society. https://www.alzheimers.org.uk/blog/laurys-mum-became-lost-in-fog-her-own-mind

Leicht, A. (2024, June 21). *10 AARP benefits all seniors should know.* CBS News. https://www.cbsnews.com/news/aarp-benefits-all-seniors-should-know/

Mapp, L. J. (2023, June 20). *Calling for backup: Why respite care is a necessary solution for caregiving burnout.* San Diego Union-Tribune; San Diego Union-Tribune. https://www.sandiegouniontribune.com/2023/06/20/calling-for-backup-why-respite-care-is-a-necessary-solution-for-caregiving-burnout/

Marie Curie. (2019). *Dementia towards the end of life.* Marie Curie. https://www.mariecurie.org.uk/professionals/palliative-care-knowledge-zone/condition-specific-short-guides/dementia

Marie Curie. (2022). *Providing spiritual care: information for healthcare professionals.* Marie Curie. https://www.mariecurie.org.uk/professionals/palliative-care-knowledge-zone/individual-needs/spiritual-care

Mayo Clinic Staff. (2021, April 29). *Alzheimer's stages: How the disease progresses.* Mayo Clinic. https://www.mayoclinic.org/diseases-conditions/alzheimers-disease/in-depth/alzheimers-stages/art-20048448

Mayo Clinic Staff. (2023). *Support groups: Make connections, get help.* Mayo Clinic. https://www.mayoclinic.org/healthy-lifestyle/stress-management/in-depth/support-groups/art-20044655

McLean, J. (2024). *10 quick and easy dysphagia diet recipes for swallowing problems.* DailyCaring. https://dailycaring.com/10-quick-and-easy-dysphagia-diet-recipes-for-swallowing-problems-5-ingredients-or-less/

Merriam-Webster. (n.d.). Dictionary. In *Merriam-Webster.com dictionary.* Retrieved September 23, 2024, from https://www.merriam-webster.com/dictionary/dictionary

NAC. (2019). *National alliance for caregiving.* Caregiving.org. https://www.caregiving.org/

National Alzheimer's and Dementia Resource Center. (n.d.-a). *Living with dementia:*

Financial planning how can I make managing my money easier? https://pblob1stor
age.blob.core.windows.net/public/nadrc/docs/Finances%20(standard).pdf

National Alzheimer's and Dementia Resource Center. (n.d.-b). *Living with dementia: planning for your care.* https://pblob1storage.blob.core.windows.net/public/nadrc/docs/Care%20Planning%20(standard).pdf

National Alzheimer's and Dementia Resource Center. (n.d.-c). *Supporting someone living with dementia in making decisions.* https://pblob1storage.blob.core.windows.net/public/nadrc/docs/Supporting%20Someone%20(standard).pdf

National Institute on Aging. (2022). *Advance care planning: Advance directives for health care.* https://www.nia.nih.gov/health/advance-care-planning/advance-care-planning-advance-directives-health-care

NIH. (2017, September 28). *Coping with grief.* NIH News in Health. https://newsin health.nih.gov/2017/10/coping-grief

A *place for everything and everything in its place.* (n.d.). The Idioms. https://www.theid ioms.com/a-place-for-everything-and-everything-in-its-place/

Porterfield, A. (2019, March 5). *Study finds a lack of adequate hydration among the elderly.* UCLA. https://newsroom.ucla.edu/releases/study-finds-a-lack-of-adequate-hydration-among-the-elderly

"Quotes for Dementia Caregivers in Need of Inspiration." ActivePro Nursing & Homecare Inc. Last modified July 10, 2018. https://www.nursehomecare.ca/site/blog/2018/07/10/homecare-services-inspirational-quotes-for-dementia-caregivers

Reisberg, B. (2019, March 28). *Clinical stages of Alzheimer's.* Fisher Center for Alzheimer's Research Foundation. https://www.alzinfo.org/understand-alzheimers/clinical-stages-of-alzheimers/

Samuels, C. (2021, September 10). *What is person-centered care for dementia?* A Place for Mom. https://www.aplaceformom.com/caregiver-resources/articles/person-centered-care-dementia

Samuels, C. (2022, February 7). *Caregiver health and stress.* A Place for Mom. https://www.aplaceformom.com/caregiver-resources/articles/caregiving-takes-toll-on-caregivers-health

Saunders, C. (n.d.). *Hospicare.* https://www.hospicare.org/wp-content/uploads/2017/07/2016-AR-POSTCARD-PP2.pdf

Sensory Direct. (2023, September 5). Sensory therapy for dementia. *Sensory Direct Blog.* https://www.sensorydirect.com/blog/the-soothing-power-of-sensory-therapy-for-dementia/

Sörensen, S., & Conwell, Y. (2011). Issues in dementia caregiving: Effects on mental and physical health, intervention strategies, and research needs. *The American Journal of Geriatric Psychiatry, 19*(6), 491–496. https://doi.org/10.1097/jgp.0b013e31821c0e6e

Sumner, K. (2016, April 22). *How to claim guardianship of an elderly parent.* Romano & Sumner, PLLC. https://romanosumner.com/blog/5-things-needed-claim-guardianship-elderly-parent/

Symptoms - Malnutrition. (2020, February 7). NHS. https://www.nhs.uk/conditions/malnutrition/symptoms/

Szlauderbach, D. (2024, January 2). *When you can no longer care for an elderly parent.* A Place for Mom. https://www.aplaceformom.com/caregiver-resources/articles/cant-be-a-caregiver

Tip sheet: How to communicate with a person living with dementia. (2022, August 3). Government of Canada. https://www.canada.ca/en/public-health/services/diseases/dementia/tip-sheet-how-communicate.html

USC School of Medicine. (2024). *A decision aid about goals of care for patients with dementia.* Palliative Care & Hospice Program. https://www.med.unc.edu/pcare/about-palliative-care/resources/goals-of-care/

Van Erdewyk, K. (2024, June 18). *Respite care: Short-term relief.* A place for mom. https://www.aplaceformom.com/caregiver-resources/articles/respite-care

Weber, M. (2019, February 19). *Alzheimer's and dementia behavior management tips.* HelpGuide.org. https://www.helpguide.org/articles/alzheimers-dementia-aging/alzheimers-behavior-management.htm

Woodruff, L. (2024, May 21). *Chasing satisfaction, not happiness, may be a healthier goal for caregivers.* AARP. https://www.aarp.org/caregiving/basics/info-2024/caregiver-satisfaction.html?intcmp=AE-CAR-BB

Yagoda, L. (2019). *National family caregiver support program.* Socialworkers.org. https://www.socialworkers.org/Practice/Aging/Aging-News/National-Family-Caregiver-Support-Program

www.ingramcontent.com/pod-product-compliance
Lightning Source LLC
Chambersburg PA
CBHW071505220526

45472CB00003B/925